THE
EATINGWELL
DIET

© Copyright 2007 by Eating Well, Inc., publisher of
EATINGWELL®, Where Good Taste Meets Good Health
823A Ferry Road, P.O. Box 1010, Charlotte, VT 05445
www.eatingwell.com

VTrim™ is a trademark of the University of Vermont and State Agricultural College ("the University") and is used with permission. The University has not reviewed, and does not warrant the effectiveness of the text in this book. This book's use or discussion of the University's VTrim™ weight-loss program services does not constitute the University's endorsement or sponsorship of a particular weight-loss approach or the appropriateness of the University's VTrim™ weight-loss program services to address a particular physical condition.

Library of Congress Cataloging-in-Publication Data has been applied for.

ISBN-13: 978-0-88150-722-5

Writer: Joyce Hendley   **Contributing Editor:** James M. Lawrence
Associate Nutrition Editor: Sylvia Geiger, M.S., R.D.

Food Editor: Jim Romanoff   **Senior Food Editor:** Jessie Price
Managing Editor: Wendy S. Ruopp   **Assistant Managing Editor:** Alesia Depot
Production Manager: Jennifer B. Brown   **Research Editor:** Anne C. Treadwell
Test Kitchen: Stacy Fraser (Test Kitchen Manager), Carolyn Malcoun (Assistant Editor),
Katie Webster (recipe developer, food stylist), Carolyn Casner (recipe tester),
Patsy Jamieson (food stylist), Susan Herr (food stylist)
Indexer: Amy Novick, BackSpace Indexing

Art Director: Michael J. Balzano   **Production Designer:** Garrett Brown
Photographer: Ken Burris   **Illustrator:** Leticia Plate

EATINGWELL MEDIA GROUP   **CEO:** Tom Witschi   **Editorial Director:** Lisa Gosselin

Front cover photograph: Paprika Shrimp & Green Bean Sauté (*page 196*)

Published by
The Countryman Press, P.O. Box 748, Woodstock, Vermont 05091
Distributed by
W.W. Norton & Company, Inc., 500 Fifth Avenue, New York, New York 10110
Printed in China by R.R. Donnelley

10 9 8 7 6 5 4 3 2 1

THE EATINGWELL DIET

INTRODUCING ——————

THE UNIVERSITY-TESTED

VTrim™ Weight-Loss Program

DR. JEAN HARVEY-BERINO, PH.D., R.D.

CHAIR OF NUTRITION AND FOOD SCIENCE, UNIVERSITY OF VERMONT

WITH JOYCE HENDLEY AND THE EDITORS OF EATINGWELL

FOREWORD BY DR. BOB ARNOT

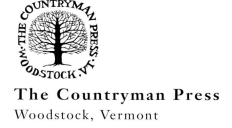

The Countryman Press
Woodstock, Vermont

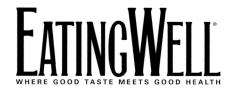

CONTENTS

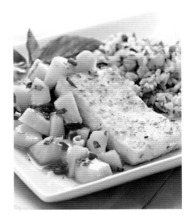

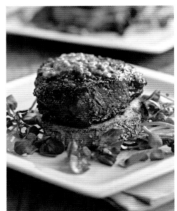

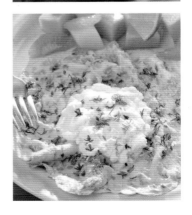

5 LIVING WELL

To make your weight loss last, move to **Step 7: Have a long-term plan.** Here, long-term maintenance strategies that work: making peace with food, preventing weight regain with a "back-on-track" strategy, countering negative thinking, and more.

6 WHAT TO EAT? 28 DAYS TO A NEW, THINNER LIFE

Four weeks of mix-and-match menus: meals and foods for healthy, permanent weight loss. You'll have the jump start to help you get thinner while working your way through the vital behavior-modification steps that will lead to a lifetime of better eating habits and instinctive self-management of weight and lifestyle.

7 EAT WELL BY COOKING WELL: 150+ EATINGWELL RECIPES

Based on the enormously popular "Healthy in a Hurry" approach developed in the EATINGWELL Vermont Test Kitchens, here are entrees and ideas for all occasions: delicious choices for everyday meals, entertaining, guilt-free desserts and snacks—all providing endless variety for different tastes and for staying easily within the bounds of *The EatingWell Diet*.

REFERENCES

An at-a-glance guide to the charts, tables and forms in the book.

ABOUT THE AUTHORS

JEAN HARVEY-BERINO, PH.D., R.D., is a professor and chair of the department of nutrition and food science at the University of Vermont. She has appeared on the *Today* Show, National Public Radio, and in numerous newspapers and magazines as an expert on the subjects of weight loss, obesity and nutrition. She is a distance runner who has completed seven marathons including Boston in 2003 and 2005. She lives with her husband and two boys, two dogs, two cats and a horse in Hinesburg, Vermont.

JOYCE HENDLEY is the Nutrition Editor of EATINGWELL Magazine, and a former Food Editor of *Weight Watchers* magazine. A frequent contributor to Weight Watchers cookbooks, she was also the writer for Sarah, the Duchess of York's best-selling *Win the Weight Game* (2000) and *The EatingWell Diabetes Cookbook* (2005). She and her family of hungry eaters live in South Burlington, Vermont.

DR. BOB ARNOT, a former chief medical editor and foreign correspondent for NBC, reports on health issues from around the world. His recent television specials, including "Doctor Danger," take him to some of the front lines in Darfur, Afghanistan and Iraq, while his CNBC series *dLife* is dedicated to Americans living with diabetes. Arnot is also the author of 11 books, the most recent *Seven Steps to Stop a Heart Attack* (2005). He is active in international relief and has served on the boards of Save the Children and the U.N. High Commission for Refugees.

EATINGWELL MAGAZINE, WHERE GOOD TASTE MEETS GOOD HEALTH, is recognized by consumers, nutritionists, journalists, and health policy makers as the most reliable, science-based source of contemporary nutrition and healthy eating information for consumers. The publication was named the winner of the James Beard Award for Food Journalism in 2003 and again in 2004, and won the Folio: Bronze Eddie Award for Epicurean Magazines in 2006. *The Essential EatingWell Cookbook* was nominated for a James Beard Award in 2005. In 2006, *The EatingWell Diabetes Cookbook* drew award nominations from both the James Beard Foundation and the International Association of Culinary Professionals. The magazine's headquarters and test kitchens are located in Charlotte, Vermont.

OTHER EATINGWELL BOOKS
(available at eatingwell.com):
The Essential EatingWell Cookbook (The Countryman Press, 2004)
ISBN-13: 978-0-88150-701-0 (softcover)

The EatingWell Diabetes Cookbook (The Countryman Press, 2005)
ISBN-13: 978-0-88150-633-4 (hardcover)

The EatingWell Healthy in a Hurry Cookbook (The Countryman Press, 2006)
ISBN-13: 978-0-88150-687-7 (hardcover)

EatingWell Serves 2 (The Countryman Press, 2006)
ISBN-13: 978-0-88150-723-2 (hardcover)

A s a longtime medical correspondent and author of books on nutrition, I've had a chance to see just about every new diet that's come out in the past two decades. In my field, it's fashionable to claim that "diets don't work." But in truth, they nearly all do—for a time. Whether they forbid carbohydrates or prescribe a mountain of fruit for breakfast, they force you to eat in a restricted way that undeniably helps get the pounds to come off.

But then they leave you stranded, without a long-term game plan. Can you really spend the rest of your days without letting an occasional baked potato pass your lips? More to the point, would you want to? And what quality of weight have you lost? Water weight? Lean muscle?

That's why I've been working for years to let people know how everyday decisions about food and exercise can transform their health. The EatingWell Diet is about this kind of transformation. It's not a diet you start, then stop when you've lost the weight. Instead, this seven-step program systematically targets the daily behaviors that lead you to gain weight—and helps you replace them with new, healthy habits that work with your lifestyle. It's a framework rather than a prescription, and one that helps you create your own strategies for eating less and moving more.

The EatingWell Diet is based on the acclaimed VTrim™ program developed at the University of Vermont, which has helped more than 1,000 people lose weight. And it works: in a multicenter study, participants in the VTrim program lost an average of 21 pounds in six months—more than twice as much weight as those in a similar study using a commercial weight-loss website program. That may not make for an attention-getting "lose 10 pounds in one week" headline, but it's the slow, steady and, most important, sustainable kind of weight loss experts recommend.

What the EatingWell plan requires of you is simple, but radical: you will commit yourself to paying attention to what you eat, how often you're active and how much you weigh. Or, in the words of VTrim founder Jean Harvey-Berino, Ph.D., you'll "track yourself to know yourself." You'll use powerful, clinically proven weight-loss tools like food diaries and activity logs.

The experience is transforming: Most people go through life in the default mode, letting the environment happen to them. They don't notice they're taking larger portions than they need or letting "other things that come up" crowd exercise out of their days. Seeing it on paper is a real wake-up call. I know. I've tried it myself.

Planning is the other cornerstone of the EatingWell approach. Working through the following pages, you'll determine the obstacles you'll face. Whether it's food-pushing relatives, rained-out walking plans or an inevitable lapse, you'll learn how to anticipate these roadblocks and confront them with your own game plan. This is the heart of successful long-term weight loss.

You'll also find helpful the 28-day menu planner and pantry-stocking tips from the kitchens of EatingWell—and especially the satisfying recipes that follow. They make those everyday choices infinitely easier, and most important, so delicious that you'll make these recipes over and over.

The EatingWell approach is about living intentionally, living well and being true to yourself. You don't go on or off it, you live it. Did I say anything about a diet?

Bob Arnot, M.D., Stowe, Vermont

READY FOR A NEW LIFE?

GETTING THIN AND STAYING THIN IS NOT AN IMPOSSIBLE DREAM

Let me guess—you've tried them all: the grapefruit diet, the grapefruit juice diet, the grapefruit *pill* diet. Or perhaps it's been the 400-calorie diet, the eat-all-you-want-as-long-as-it's (protein, rice, bread, steak, name-your-food-any-food) diet. It could have been one of the many no-diet diets. Maybe you've eaten low-fat or high-fat, high-carb or low-carb, high-fiber or even low-fiber. It's possible you've tried to eat like Miami socialites, Japanese fishermen, svelte French women, or even Neanderthal hunters. It could be that you've done the exercise clubs, the video workout routines, or the plastic-wrap spot-reducing plans. They might even have worked… until they didn't.

Even as myriad new weight-loss schemes appear, most of us already know the verdict: diets don't work. In the vast majority of cases, people drop out of the diet within weeks and regain the weight. A significant percentage rebound from a diet to gain even more weight than they started with. You are probably suspicious of the word "diet," and I don't blame you.

That's why we're going to give you a plan—much more than a weight-loss diet—where the odds of success, once you start, are truly in your favor.

Fad Diet Radar

We've all fallen victim to quirky (and quacky) diet and exercise plans over the years. Any diet that promises "quick and easy" weight loss should raise a big red flag. Suspect a fad that's more promise than substance if the diet plan says you must:

- Avoid an entire food group or a specific food

- Take pills or supplements (especially if the diet "won't work" without them)

- Eat certain foods because they'll "cure" a disease

- Avoid certain foods because they'll "cause" a disease

- Eat foods only at certain times or in specific combinations

- Eat only foods prepared in a certain way

A weight-loss diet, by definition, is temporary—something you're meant to go on, then off. You're told what to eat and when to eat it—often based on some complicated scientific rationale that involves, say, hormone fluctuations, metabolic manipulations or maybe the phases of the moon. In truth, there are many approaches to eating and just as many exercise plans that can help you lose weight. There is no one correct way to go about it, although there are plenty of wrong methods. You can easily find an array of new diets on the supermarket tabloid rack every week—and they all sound so fast and so, so easy. So what can we offer that you haven't tried already?

In 15 years of weight-loss research and working with thousands of people trying to get trimmer and feel healthier, I have come to find that almost everyone knows the truth: to lose the weight, we need to eat less and move more. This book is about the missing link: **how to do it**.

How do you start eating better foods, how do you stop skipping breakfast, how do you resist all those fast-food lunches, how you start a walking program and stick with it?

Our focus is on behavior change—permanent behavior change. It's only through a systematic shaping of everyday common behaviors that you will be able to break old habits and learn new ones. Drinking grapefruit juice until you scream is a behavior change, of course, but not the kind that you will sustain for very long.

Here's how the behavioral approach we have developed at the University of Vermont differs from traditional diet strategy: Say you get a lot of your calories at night, after dinner in front of the TV. A typical "diet" solution would be to substitute carrot sticks for the chips and ice cream you'd normally snack on. That might work for a time, but it doesn't break the behavior of eating in front of the TV. In this book, we'll show you how to change the behavior that got you to the weight gain in the first place—not just help you learn to love carrots.

HOW DID WE GET HERE ANYWAY?

There is an almost maniacal focus on the problem of weight in this country. Given the amount of time and energy the media spend ruminating about our waistlines, one would think we should all be uniformly thin. So why are we one of the fattest countries on earth? More people are heavy—and more heavy people are heavier than ever before. The problem is all too real, and if you are struggling with your weight, you are far from alone.

A lot has to do with our highly industrialized society: In the past 50 years there has been an unprecedented transformation to new technologies designed to save us time and energy. We have garage door openers, electric clothes dryers, power toothbrushes, even gizmos that warm up our cars in winter so we don't have to go outside and scrape off the ice. If there are ways to save steps, avoid lifting, stretching, bending or moving, inventors have been there, done that or are fixing things as we speak. There are remote controls for everything, and computers do almost all the legwork for us. I don't even have to flip the light switch in my office when I enter or leave; it's done automatically with a sensing device.

Individually all these labor-saving devices aren't responsible for that collective spare tire around society's middle, but they do have a bigger cumulative impact. Consider that if you walk just two minutes less than you normally do each day, you could gain a pound of fat over the course of a year. Two minutes! So little things do add up over time, and all the conveniences of modern life that we've grown accustomed to are working against staying at a healthy weight.

Combine this trend with the supersizing of modern food portions and you have the perfect storm for weight gain: We have access to more calories—and more relatively cheap calories— now than at any other time in our history. And there are more creative marketing techniques designed to seduce us into buying this food, including giant-portioned value meals and economy-size packages, appetite-triggering advertising campaigns—and lots and lots of sugary drinks. How many soda machines and soda-hawking billboards did you pass today?

The 6.5-ounce green-glass Coke bottle many of us remember from our childhoods is now just a quaint collector's item, shunted aside by the popular 20-ounce size soda, along with multi-liter jumbo jugs and all manner of Big Gulping, Super Slugging, Bottomless Guzzling vats of high-calorie pop. And the phenomenon holds true throughout the national menu: an average muffin has ballooned from about 200 calories two decades ago to more than 500 today; a serving of spaghetti and meatballs has more than doubled from an average of 500 calories to more than 1,000 and a serving of fries that we once thought just right has been mounded up from 200 calories in the early 1970s to more than 600 calories today.

We are also eating out more often, and in most places we're served "single" portions that could feed a small country. It's gotten so prevalent that we don't even notice when a portion is overly hefty. Studies show that even food and nutrition professionals have trouble accurately judging portion sizes or estimating calorie counts when they encounter foods prepared outside the home.

DROPPING OUT, GETTING TRIM

These days, if you want to eat right and live a healthy lifestyle, you wind up being part of the counterculture, opting out of the All-American ways of doing things. We often tell our weight-loss program participants that it's like being a salmon swimming upstream, fighting the current that tries to sweep you toward the 24-hour all-you-can-eat buffet. Sadly, the buffet current is nearly as strong as the tide that pulls you onto the couch every night.

It now takes a conscious effort to maintain a healthy lifestyle as a part of mainstream America. We value productivity, efficiency and achievement. Because of this, we work long hours and microwave meals in pouches when we get home. We obsess about food but we don't value it; what we value is a value. Why buy a single-serving bag of pretzels when you can get a huge tub of them at a bulk price? Why not supersize when it only costs pennies more? Top the burger with bacon, stuff the pizza dough with extra cheese, some whipped cream on the cappuccino? Why not?

Because we all have to live in this so-called "obesigenic" environment in which many factors conspire to fuel the human genetic tendency to gain weight, I'm convinced that no weight-loss program can truly succeed unless it tackles behavioral change. We develop eating behaviors based on what we are familiar with, what we like and what works in the moment. To succeed, we need to reverse the urgings of marketers to eat more, eat more often, and eat more decadent foods while avoiding steps and physical labor whenever possible. Changing those behaviors is exceedingly hard, but it can be done. I see it happen all the time.

WEIGHT LOSS YOU CAN SUSTAIN

Contrary to popular belief, it *is* possible to lose weight and keep it off. Just ask anyone enrolled in the National Weight Control Registry (http://www.nwcr.ws/). In order to be a member of the NWCR you must have lost at least 30 pounds and kept it off for a year. It sounds daunting, but most of the 5,000-plus NWCR members have actually lost an average of 60 pounds, and kept it off for over five years.

Clearly none of them would ever say that losing weight is easy—and I'll be honest: there is no magic solution. No pills, powders, potions or tropical juice blends will melt fat. The registry members report eating a diet that's moderate in calories and fat, and they get plenty of regular exercise. They have lost weight through a variety of methods; one size doesn't fit all. However, despite their differences, they have all managed to *change their behavior* in meaningful ways in order to achieve a lower, healthier weight that's sustainable.

> ❝ If you have made mistakes, even serious ones, there is always another chance for you. What we call failure is not the falling down but the staying down. ❞
>
> MARY PICKFORD, ACTRESS

What's more, they report that keeping weight off gets easier over time. Their healthy habits—once consciously learned—have now become instincts, so sticking with them isn't such an effort. If they can do it, you can too.

I can say with confidence that, if you have picked up this book, you have what you need to succeed at losing weight. I've been researching weight management for over 15 years, and this book contains the best of what I and others have learned about the techniques and strategies that promote long-term weight loss and maintenance.

THE VTRIM PHENOMENON

Back in 2002, my colleagues and I were frustrated. More Americans were overweight or obese than ever, while at the same time, there seemed to be thousands of weight-loss programs, all promising glowing success. But whether the diets focused on eating strictly low-fat or high protein or all-cabbage soup, none of them seemed to be very effective in the long run.

But we knew from our own research, and that of other national and international behavioral strategists, that there were plenty of workable strategies that could make weight loss not only possible, but sustainable. What was needed was a comprehensive plan that put all the best pieces together. That's when we created VTrim at the University of Vermont.

The VTrim program consists of 24 weekly weight-management lessons that focus on the behavioral approach to weight loss, delivered in group meetings—either online or in person—by Nutrition and Behavior Modification professionals. Participants in the program (we call them VTrimmers) learn the basics of weight management: eating less and moving more—while tracking their eating and activity patterns as well as tackling the emotions and situations that trigger them to overeat. Our aim is that

> **" Let your head be more than a funnel to your stomach. "**
> GERMAN PROVERB

when they complete the program, they've got what they need to keep their weight on track for life—and that we never need to see them again. (Unlike a commercial diet program, we don't profit from members who relapse, regain and then return for another round of dieting.)

In the four years since VTrim began, over 1,000 VTrimmers have successfully completed the program and collectively lost thousands of pounds. (You'll hear some of their stories, and learn from their struggles and successes, throughout this book.) And lose weight they do: an average of about 21 pounds in six months, whether they participate in online or group meetings. Keep in mind that that figure just represents an average; while some VTrimmers enter the program with just 15 to 20 pounds to lose, many lose in the neighborhood of 50 pounds-plus. In fact, when compared head-to-head with participants in a commercial online weight-loss program, VTrimmers lost more than twice as much weight. Even more significant: they were better able to maintain that weight loss one year later than the other group. And they're not likely to put those pounds back on again, because they've mastered lifetime weight-management skills.

All the key elements of the VTrim lessons are included in this book, reconfigured for you to follow on your own in your own home. We've found that six months is a realistic time frame to fully assimilate information about weight loss and to be able to apply it. Remember, it's not a race—it's a lifetime commitment to a healthy lifestyle, so we encourage you to think in the long term too.

While you'll personalize our approach to fit your life, some element of each program component will speak

> **" Life itself is the proper binge. "**
>
> JULIA CHILD

to you. For example, you may be someone who has little problem avoiding rich gooey desserts, but just can't seem to find a way to exercise. Or you may have no problem controlling your food intake from 9 to 5, but look out after the sun goes down! Everyone has different eating and exercise issues, but the techniques for solving them have common components.

In each chapter, we've outlined many different strategies to help you be successful. You'll start by learning key skills of self-coaching: how to keep track of your eating and exercise behaviors. Next, we'll focus on how to make good food choices and sensible portion sizes—and how to start and sustain an exercise program. Later, you'll discover proven strategies for controlling your environment to make it more conducive to a healthy lifestyle, as well as how to maintain motivation and get back on track when you've "fallen off the wagon" (don't worry, everyone does at some point). And, once you've lost the weight, we'll help you plan a lifetime strategy for maintaining your success. Each program component results from cutting-edge research, put into practice in real people's lives.

EATING WELL FOR LIFE

Even though you'll need to cut back on calories to lose weight, eating (as one of my colleagues often says) should always be more than just "filling up the tank." That's why a key section of this book takes the VTrim program one step beyond—with great food. We've collaborated with our neighbors at EATINGWELL, the premier magazine of food and health. The recipes, menus, eating and cooking tips and advice for stocking your pantry that EATINGWELL provides are all designed to make it easier than ever for you to eat deliciously, seasonally and healthfully.

And, if you need an extra boost to help get you started on the path to losing weight, check out the 28 days of menus, recipes and inspirational tips in Chapter 6. Use the menus as you see fit, mixing and matching, or repeating entrees if you like, for as long as you like: you'll pick up a lot of wisdom about meal patterns, portion sizes, and calorie counts that can get you "in the groove" for changing your own meal-planning and eating behavior. We've done the calorie counting and nutritional balancing for you. You don't have to use the menus, but they're a terrific resource.

Hard-Wired for the Clean Plate Club

When you're faced with that trough of pasta at your favorite Italian restaurant, why is it so hard to avoid cleaning your plate, even after reaching a fully stuffed state? Blame biological mechanisms, which kick in as soon as you see and smell the lasagna.

We are all born with an instinctive desire to seek out high-calorie food—and to eat as much of it as possible when we have access to it. We're also driven to seek dietary variety. Why? It makes sense from a biological perspective: How often did a caveman get to fell a woolly mammoth? When he got one, his survival depended on eating a lot of it, *and fast*, before it spoiled; he never knew when another mammoth might cross his path. And in order to get enough nutrients to survive, he had to learn to eat more than just mammoth meat.

Obviously, this biologic strategy worked: our species survived, even though the mammoth is long extinct. But unfortunately, while our genetics are designed to manage the occasional mammoth, they have not adapted to a constantly available food supply—not to mention the frequent 32-ounce cola. Studies by Brian Wansink at Cornell University and Barbara Rolls at Penn State have consistently found that we eat more when served larger portions. It doesn't even matter if the food is good or bad. It's just human nature to clean the plate.

The fusion of EATINGWELL's wonderfully satisfying foods with the VTrim program has brought us into new, exciting territory. After all, not long ago behavioral weight-control experts like me believed it was counterproductive to tell weight-loss-program participants what to eat. Our goal was to encourage folks to make permanent changes in their behavior, so we reasoned that no one could ever learn how to eat if they were being told exactly what to put in their mouths for breakfast, lunch and dinner. Moreover, we worried that our prescriptions might not incorporate someone's favorite foods or be adaptable to family dining situations, and thus wouldn't be effective for making lasting dietary changes. In other words, our prescriptions would resemble a DIET—and we all know what kind of track record weight-loss diets have.

Well, it turned out we were wrong. In fact, people seem to lose more weight with some guidance about which foods to choose—and with menus, recipes and grocery lists that help take the guesswork out of food. It also makes sense from a behavioral perspective: knowing what to eat helps limit your choices in the grocery store, so it helps you control your eating environment. (With the average supermarket stocking over 45,000 items, it's no wonder we need help!)

With both EATINGWELL and VTrim in your corner, you don't need to be a star chef—or a chef at all!—to be able to make healthy, appealing, calorie-smart meals for yourself and your family.

We won't promise you 10 pounds in 10 days—you can find that plan on late-night TV. Rather, we encourage a slow, reasonable weight loss of 1 to 2 pounds a week. Weight loss faster than this is likely not fat but muscle and water weight. Remember, the average weight loss for VTrimmers over six months is 21 pounds; it's not about what you are willing to put up with in the short term, it's about how you want to live in the long term. Veteran dieters can tell how rapid weight loss virtually always comes back (often with a vengeance), and they also talk about the euphoria of finally achieving sustainable, steady week-in-week-out weight loss with a science-based plan.

Let's take the first step, by making sure you're ready for the journey.

> "I think the word that comes to mind to me over and over again is that this is just such a doable program. I don't think of it at all as a diet. I think of it as just my life now…I feel like I can keep living my life. I'm a person who really enjoys food and I'm able to incorporate that, and I never feel like I don't get enough to eat or something like that.
>
> "The way the program is structured, it seems to prepare you for the variability of life really well."
>
> —**Gail**, 53 (50 pounds lost)

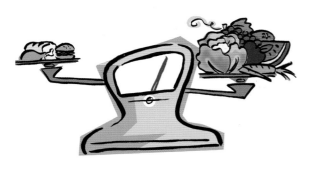

STEP 1: MAKE SURE YOU'RE READY FOR CHANGE

Of course you want to lose weight—that's why you are reading this—but in order to make a life plan you can stick with, you must be ready—*truly ready*—to make the commitment. Losing weight will take some time and effort, and it will require you to make some sacrifices (if it were easy, everyone would be thin!). But as our pool of successful "losers" can confirm, the results can truly justify the journey. The first step is to make sure you're ready to get started.

Before you go any further in this book, take a few minutes now to assess what you'll gain from losing weight, considering your lifestyle now and in the future. Better health, more energy? Feeling better, more confident in your clothes? Being more attractive to a partner—or a potential partner? List as many as you can think of on the worksheet on the next page. Then, list the sacrifices you expect you'll have to make, being as honest with yourself as possible. Finding a window of time in each day to take a walk might seem daunting, for example.

Now, look at your list and weigh the advantages and disadvantages. Chances are, one side will be a lot longer than the other, showing you a clear path to the right decision. You might also decide that some factors have greater importance than the others. For example, Jenna, a 51-year-old woman with hypertension, was urged by her doctor to lose weight to help control her blood pressure. That factor made all the disadvantages she listed ("will have to get up an hour earlier to exercise," "don't want to ask for special foods at parties, restaurants,") seem relatively unimportant.

If you've really given it some thought and the "minus" side is more substantial than the "plus" side, you might want to reconsider starting the program now. If you're not wholeheartedly committed, your chances of succeeding are much lower. And we *know* you don't want to fail at another weight-loss effort. Consider putting the plan aside for now, and repeating this exercise in a few weeks. Your answers might be quite different then.

Take Paulette, who just started a new, stressful job that required her to put in many extra hours to bring herself to the same level as her co-workers. Although she was eager to have a new, slimmer identity to match her new career, the thought of planning and shopping for meals and finding time for exercise just sounded like too much to handle. So she decided to put off trying to lose weight until she felt more in control of her time.

Was Paulette a "quitter"? Far from it. In fact, by waiting until she had the time and resources to commit to losing weight, Paulette *avoided* being a quitter who might have gone on to a failed weight-loss attempt, leaving her even more unhappy, and maybe even heavier, than before. When she finally decided the time was right a few months later, she greatly improved her chances of success in losing the weight, once and for all.

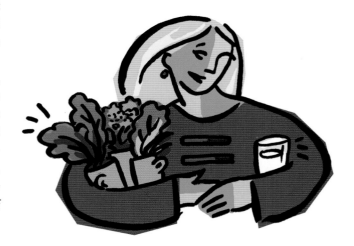

CHECK-IN: PLUSES AND MINUSES OF LOSING WEIGHT NOW

PLUS
+

WHAT I'LL GET BY LOSING WEIGHT:

_____
_____
_____
_____
_____
_____
_____
_____
_____
_____
_____
_____
_____
_____
_____
_____
_____
_____
_____
_____
_____

MINUS
—

WHAT I'LL GIVE UP:

_____
_____
_____
_____
_____
_____
_____
_____
_____
_____
_____
_____
_____
_____
_____
_____
_____
_____
_____
_____
_____

CHAPTER 1

BECOME YOUR OWN WEIGHT COACH

TAKE CHARGE: WITH THESE ESSENTIAL TOOLS

Wouldn't it be wonderful to have a personal weight manager—someone to coach you through the weight-loss process, someone to custom-tailor an eating and exercise plan that is just right for you? Someone who can help keep you on track, monitor your progress, and give you positive encouragement just when you feel your motivation flagging? The kind of personal coach that Hollywood glitterati rely on, and pay top dollar for?

Truth be told, you don't need to hire anyone. Ultimately, you have the power within yourself to become your own personal coach. Your own mind is an incredibly potent weight-loss tool, especially when you've mastered a few simple techniques of behavior modification, which we'll detail throughout this book. (Of course, your mind can also work in the opposite direction, helping you to *gain* weight. Much of what you'll learn is how to "deprogram" these unhealthy thought patterns.) Once you've aligned your thinking toward the goal of losing weight, you'll have the skills you need to coach yourself through your own weight-loss journey. After all, who knows you better than you?

Let's begin, as any personal coach would, with a thorough assessment of where you are now, and where you'd like to be—and use that information to set your personal goals. Then, we'll introduce a few self-coaching tools that are fundamental to the behavioral approach to weight loss.

> " A goal is created three times. First as a mental picture. Second, when written down to add clarity and dimension. And third, when you take action towards its achievement. "
>
> GARY RYAN BLAIR, "THE GOALS GUY"

WEIGHING IN

Now that you've made a commitment to lose weight, it's time to take stock. What is your weight now, and how far is it from where you'd like it to be?

Many of us have an idea of what we'd like to weigh, and usually it's based on notions that are long on idealism and short on reality. If you're 45, it's probably not realistic to think you can get back to your high school weight. Trying to achieve fashion-model thinness is probably a waste of energy, too, since most top models are woefully underweight by any standard. So what is a sensible weight for you?

Rather than focusing on a single, arbitrary number of pounds, focus instead on finding a healthy weight range—that is, a weight that's associated with a longer, healthier life and lower risk of the diseases linked to being overweight (high blood pressure, stroke, heart disease, diabetes and others). Most experts determine healthy-weight ranges with a calculation that takes both weight and height into account to give you a single number called a Body Mass Index (BMI) value.

The BMI is a pretty reliable way to measure your health outlook; in general, the lower your BMI, the lower your risks of health problems related to your weight. But a BMI value doesn't give you the whole picture. For starters, it's not a reliable measurement for pregnant or breastfeeding women, who need to have larger fat stores to support a growing baby or to produce milk. The BMI is downright misleading for some bodybuilders or competitive athletes, too: since muscle is denser than fat, a well-muscled body may register as "obese" on the BMI scale.

For all these reasons, most experts also take a second measurement in addition to the BMI: waist size. Why the waist? Studies show that people who have more fat around their abdomens tend to have greater risks of problems like heart disease and diabetes—so knowing what the tape tells you about your waist circumference can help determine your overall health prognosis.

In general, health problems increase when a waist measurement—not your belt size, by the way—is greater than 40 inches for men and 35 inches for women. So, if your BMI puts you in a higher risk category, having a waist size above those numbers raises your level of risk even higher and adds to the list of reasons you would want to lose weight.

Turn to the table on page 236 to determine your own BMI value. You'll need to weigh yourself and measure your height, then write your calculations on the Goal-Setting Worksheet on page 18. Next, measure your waist with a tape measure, at belly-button level, and record it in the space provided.

> **"A goal properly set is halfway reached."**
>
> ABRAHAM LINCOLN

Example: Jeff, who is 6 feet (72 inches) tall and weighs 211 pounds, calculated his BMI between 29 (the value at 208 pounds) and 30 (the value at 215 pounds), putting him just below the border of the "high risk" category. But because he measured his waist at 40 inches exactly, he considers himself squarely in high-risk territory. "That's an extra incentive for me to get a handle on my weight now."

Now, use the chart that follows to determine where you are on the risk scale.

If your BMI is:	Your health risk profile is:
Below 25	IDEAL. You probably don't need to lose weight for health reasons, though it might boost your self-esteem and confidence.
25 - 29.9	MODERATE. Your chance of developing heart disease, diabetes and other diseases associated with excess weight is higher, especially at the higher numbers in this range. Losing some weight can help you feel great now—and it can also prevent you from sliding into a higher risk category later on. **Waist size over 40" (men) or 35" (women)?** Your risk of health problems is increased, but weight loss can bring your numbers into a healthier range.
30 & higher	HIGH RISK. Officially categorized as "obese," you might already be facing some health issues related to your weight. But take heart: you'll see the most dramatic effects on your health and well-being as the weight comes off. **Waist size over 40" (men) or 35" (women)?** With the help of your doctor, make a commitment to lose some weight—your health and well-being depend on it.

GOAL-SETTING WORKSHEET

DATE: _____

MY WEIGHT: _____

MY BMI: _____

MY WAIST SIZE: _____

MY LONG-TERM WEIGHT-LOSS GOAL

For my height, a weight of _____ will put me within a healthy BMI range.
I will need to lose _____ pounds.

MY STARTING GOAL

To lose 10% of my weight, I will need to lose _____ pounds.

MY WEIGHT-MAINTENANCE NUMBER

My weight _____ pounds x 12 = _____ calories/day

MY DAILY CALORIE GOAL

_____ weight-maintenance number

_____ subtract 500 or 1,000 calories

_____ equals calories/day

STEP 2: SET YOUR GOALS

This brings you to the next step of your weight loss journey: deciding what kind of weight loss makes sense for you.

The big picture. Start by sketching out an ultimate, long-term goal. For a rough guide, you can use the BMI table on page 236. After you've located your height on the left side of the table, follow it across until you reach the weight that would put you in a healthy BMI range (we recommend a target BMI of 24). Subtract that weight from your current weight to determine how many pounds you'd need to lose, then record your answers on Goal Setting Worksheet, page 18.

For Jeff's height of 6 feet, a weight of 172 pounds will put him at a healthy weight range, with a BMI of 24.

He will need to lose:

$$\begin{array}{r} 211 \text{ pounds} \\ - 172 \text{ pounds} \\ \hline 39 \text{ pounds} \end{array}$$

If that number seems impossibly large, don't panic—remember, you're looking at the big picture with a long-term goal. At the safe, slow rate of weight loss we recommend—1 to 2 pounds per week—it could take you some time to get there. (Jeff calculates it will take him at least 20 weeks, or about five months.) And it should! After all, we are talking about permanent life change, not a quick fix.

The power of 10. But you don't have to reach your ultimate weight goal to see benefits in your health status and in how you look and feel. In fact, losing just 10 percent of your body weight—just 17 pounds, if you weigh 170—can give you terrific results in all those areas. Studies show that for most people, a 10 percent weight loss can lower blood pressure and cholesterol numbers, and even reduce your risks of developing diabetes if your blood-sugar levels are "borderline" high. And that's not to mention the unscientific benefits: just imagine how your clothes will fit, how people will notice your new, trimmer look, and the boost in your confidence and energy levels. One recent study also suggests that it may even improve your sex life: Duke University researchers found that when a group of very obese men and women lost approximately 11 percent of their body weight, their sexual quality of life improved significantly—including their feelings of sexual attractiveness and desire.

Too Fast? Too Slow?

Wonderful as it may sound, losing weight rapidly—more than 3 pounds a week—isn't healthy in the long term. At that rate, you're not only burning off fat, you're starting to lose lean muscle tissue, too—and that can slow down the rate at which you burn calories off, making it paradoxically harder to lose pounds.

So if you're losing more than 3 pounds a week for more than three weeks in a row, it's time to raise your calorie goal. Try adding an extra serving or two of whole grains or an extra piece of fruit each day (about 75-100 calories each), until your weight loss drops into the healthy 1-2 pound range.

Likewise, if you're not losing a pound or more per week, you might need to dial down your calorie goal a little (as long as it doesn't go below 1,200 calories/day). Try cutting out a discretionary item first—say, a serving of (non-whole-grain) starch. For an easier, more positive-sounding fix, you could increase your activity level so you burn more calories (more about that in Chapter 3).

A 10 percent weight loss, then, is a great starting goal—and, more important, it's within your reach, no matter where you're starting out. To calculate, just divide your current weight by 10, round it up or down to the nearest whole number, and enter it as your "Starting Goal" on the Goal-Setting Worksheet. Now, you've got a doable target—and when you achieve it, you'll have a lot to celebrate!

For Jeff's current weight of 211 pounds:
211/10 = 21.1
Round down to 21

Jeff's starting goal: 21 pounds

> **" I'm not overweight. I'm just nine inches too short. "**
> SHELLEY WINTERS, ACTRESS

A BALANCING ACT: HOW CALORIES AFFECT YOUR WEIGHT

We've all seen the pop-diet ads: *Never Count Calories Again!*, but the fact is that we can't talk about weight loss without talking about calories. Without doubt, one of the leading causes of overweight is not knowing—or not wanting to know—how many calories we consume in a day.

But what exactly are calories, and why do they matter? Calories are simply the unit we use to measure the amount of energy supplied by food, and the amount burned by activity. If the number of calories you eat equals the number of calories you burn through exercise, your weight stays the same; this is called "energy balance."

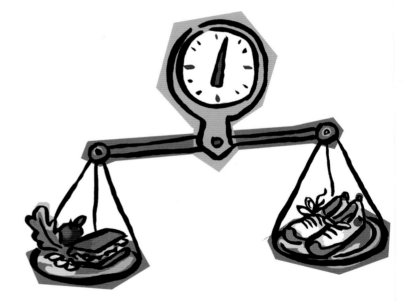

If you eat more calories than you burn, you have a calorie surplus. Your body, in its wisdom, stores those extra calories in case they're needed later— say, in a famine. It packs those calories into highly efficient storage units that contain 3,500 calories of stored energy in every pound. (You might know those storage units by their more common name: fat.) The ultimate result: You put on fat, and gain weight.

So to lose weight, you need to create a *negative* energy balance, in the opposite direction, by:

> **decreasing the calories you take in (eating less)**
> *and/or*
> **increasing the calories you burn (exercising more).**

The best, most effective method is to do both.

To lose one pound, then, you need to create a negative energy balance of 3,500 calories—the amount stored in one pound of fat. Take the math a step further, and you'll see that cutting 500 calories from what you eat each day will add up to 3,500 calories per week. That should result in a weight loss of about 1 pound per week. Likewise, a deficit of 1,000 calories per day will add up to 2 pounds of weight loss per week.

500 fewer calories per day x 7 days = 3,500 fewer calories per week = about 1 pound lost

1,000 fewer calories per day x 7 days = 7,000 fewer calories per week = about 2 pounds lost

HOW MANY CALORIES DO YOU NEED?

Let's start by figuring out how many calories you actually need just to keep your weight the way it is now (that is, in energy balance). This amount depends on your size, how active you are and your *metabolic rate*—the amount of calories your body needs for basic functions like breathing. Many formulas take all these factors into account, but can get quite complicated.

We prefer a method that is utterly simple: Multiply your weight in pounds times 12 to get your weight maintenance number, and enter it on the Goal-Setting Worksheet (*page 18*). Assuming your weight has been stable, this gives you a good estimate of the amount of calories you have been eating to maintain your weight.

> When you hear people say "cut your calories," what does that mean? Until I followed this program, I never knew how it worked. Diet programs will tell you to eat 1,200 calories per day, but they don't give you the context or show you how to figure out how many calories you're currently eating. It's so simple and so meaningful.
>
> —**Jan**, 47 (58 pounds lost)

> **"You got to be careful if you don't know where you're going, because you might not get there."**
>
> YOGI BERRA

Sarah, who weighs 150 pounds, needs 1,800 daily calories per day to maintain her weight.

(150 x 12 = 1,800-calorie weight-maintenance number)

Jeff, who weighs 211 pounds, needs 2,532 daily calories to keep his weight steady.

(211 x 12 = 2,532-calorie weight-maintenance number)

YOUR CALORIE CALCULATION FOR LOSING WEIGHT

Now that you know the number of calories that will keep your weight steady, you can subtract calories from that daily total to produce a weight loss at the safe rate of 1 to 2 pounds per week:

Either 500 calories, for an approximate 1-pound weekly weight loss
or
1,000 calories for an approximate 2-pound weekly weight loss

NOTE: The lowest calorie goal for this program is 1,200 calories. Below that amount of calories, it's hard to meet your daily nutrition requirements. So, if your calorie goal falls below 1,200 calories, set it at 1,200. You'll still lose weight!

WHY GOALS ARE GOLDEN

Every coach knows how important goals are. They provide something to aim for—and a way of measuring your progress. There's nothing more motivating than a sense of accomplishment, so with every goal you achieve, you create more positive momentum on your weight-loss journey. We want you to set plenty of goals regularly, and we'll work more specifically on how to do that in future chapters.

You'll get the most out of your goals if you keep the following tips in mind:

HAVE BOTH SHORT- AND LONG-TERM GOALS. Long-term goals provide a sense of purpose and keep you oriented in the right direction. They work best if they're not so far in the future that they seem unattainable: ideally, six months or up to one year. Short-term goals focus on a more immediate time frame, such as "this week" or "this month." They move you toward your larger goals and give you feedback that your efforts are paying off.

BE REALISTIC. Setting an impossible goal—say, "I'll never eat fast food again"—is self-defeating, as only a superhuman could reach it. And an unachievable goal sets you up for failure, which can send your thoughts in a devastating tailspin ("I broke my promise to myself, so why not just give up altogether?"). Focus instead on a goal you know you can attain with some effort—or break a large goal into smaller, more manageable steps. A more realistic approach to the fast-food goal might be: "I'll cut down on fast-food meals to just twice a month."

CHOOSE SPECIFIC AND MEASURABLE GOALS. Being clear about your goal gives you a better chance of understanding when you've reached it. Tie your goal to a specific action if you can: Rather than saying "I'll eat vegetables more often," try "I'll eat at least one serving of vegetables at lunch and one at dinner every day this week."

REWARD YOURSELF. As you reach your goals, make sure you acknowledge your achievement with a reward. This tangible recognition of "closure" on your goal is powerfully motivating, so don't skip it! Your reward doesn't have to be expensive, but it should be something meaningful to you. Think of something that is not food-related: Rent or go to a movie, schedule a massage, buy yourself a book, some music or a flattering piece of clothing you've had your eye on. For many of us, time for ourselves is the most luxurious gift of all. How about a 10-minute phone call to a long-missed friend, or a half-hour undisturbed soak in the bathtub?

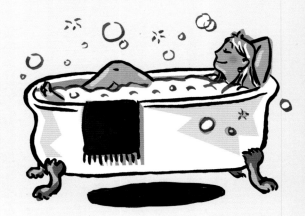

REVISE GOALS WHEN YOU NEED TO. Once you've reached a goal, set a new one, so that you continue to keep yourself challenged and motivated. If your goal was to work up to walking a mile three times a week, set the bar a little higher—say, a mile and a quarter.

Sarah wants to lose 2 pounds per week:

Weight maintenance number: 1,800

                              −1,000

                      = **800** **calories/day**—This is too low to support good nutrition, so Sarah's daily calorie goal is 1,200 calories/day.

Jeff wants to lose 2 pounds per week too:

Weight maintenance number: 2,532

                              −1,000

                      = **1,532** **calories/day**—Jeff's Daily Calorie Goal

June, who weighs 182 pounds, votes for a 500 daily calorie-cutting goal ("More sounds too hard!"):

Weight maintenance number: 2,184

                              −500

                      = **1,684** **calories/day**—June's Daily Calorie Goal

Now, calculate *your* daily calorie goal and enter it on the goal-setting worksheet.

STEP 3: TRACK YOURSELF

Now that you know where you stand weight-wise, it's time to introduce the concept of behavior modification that makes this program work: self-tracking. Simply put, self-tracking is keeping track of the actions that affect your weight—namely, your eating and exercise habits—by writing them down. In doing so, you have a record of your behavior over time.

It begins with keeping a food diary: a place to record all the foods you eat, how much you eat and when you eat, as well as a tally of the calories each item contributes. In the EATINGWELL Food Diary (*see page 24 for a sample page*), there's also space to jot down thoughts and feelings, which can clue you in to the thought patterns that contribute to your eating habits.

Be ready for a sobering experience. In the VTrim program, there are many highly educated, professional people who discover that they had no idea of how many calories they were eating in a typical day.

Start keeping a food diary today, and you're already on your way to losing weight. In fact, you might lose weight even if you make no other changes. How? Being more self-aware helps tip you off to behaviors (and calories) that contribute to weight gain, and helps you break bad habits. By writing something down, you become accountable for it, you have evidence of your behavior. That in itself is incredibly motivating for most people. It's not just about changing your food choices, it's about recognizing the behaviors that lead to problem food choices. Think of Pinocchio: he couldn't break the habit of lying, until each lie made his nose grow longer. With the evidence right under our noses, making better choices each day gets easier and easier. That's what keeping a food diary can do for you.

"At first the VTrim people said, 'Don't do anything. Just do the diary. Write everything down, figure it out, and be completely honest.'

"That's an eye opener because once you start looking at the things you're used to eating, you realize two things: one is that your portion size has gone through the roof over the years. The second is the calorie-density of foods that you select...it's so easy to eat very, very calorie-dense food."

—**John**, 50 (75 pounds lost)

Here's how a typical day's diary page might look, if you've already had your lunch by now:

SAMPLE FOOD DIARY PAGE

TIME	PORTION	FOOD/ BEVERAGE DESCRIPTION	CALORIES	NOTES
7:15	2-oz.	Bagel	154	
	1 Tbsp.	Low-fat cream cheese	35	
	½ cup	Orange juice	56	
10:50	3-inch	Blueberry Danish	335	Couldn't resist coffee cart—felt guilty
1:30		Deli sandwich:		Starving!
	2 slices	Rye bread	140	
	3 oz.	Ham, extra-lean	99	
	2 slices	Tomato and lettuce	5	
	1 Tbsp.	Mayonnaise	99	
	2-oz. bag	Baked sour cream & onion chips	240	
	12-oz.	Diet cola	0	

STARTING YOUR FOOD DIARY

Turn to page 237 for a blank food-diary page, make a copy, and start writing down everything you eat and drink today. A few ground rules:

Keep it handy. Take your food diary with you everywhere, so it's always at the ready whenever an eating opportunity presents itself (say, that sliver of cake at a surprise office birthday celebration). For convenience, you can also use a small notepad to write down what you eat, then enter the list in your diary later.

Write it right after you bite it. That way, you won't forget anything, especially quantities. Don't forget condiments, like that pat of butter on your green beans. Be sure to include those "incidental" nibbles that are notoriously easy to overlook—like that last quarter of a grilled-cheese sandwich you polished off when your child left it on her plate, or that mini candy bar from the jar on your co-worker's desk.

"Food diaries...that's the key to this. When people in our group reported that they weren't losing weight, it usually turned out that they hadn't been writing everything down. Some people don't write it down because they know they're 'cheating.' But being an engineer, I see it differently. If you know the formula, it's only going to work if you do it right."

—**David**, 49 (76 pounds lost)

Be specific. Record the type and amount of food in as much detail as possible, especially portion sizes; list "10 crackers," rather than "a handful," or "2 cups popcorn" rather than "small bowl." (For quick ways to help you "eyeball" portion sizes, see Chapter 2.)

Record calories. Use the calorie charts in the back of this book, starting on page 240, to look up the calorie value of the foods and drinks you've had today, making sure to adjust for the portion size. For example, if that portion of ham in your sandwich at lunch was larger than the 1-ounce-slice serving listed in the calorie guide, make sure to adjust the calories accordingly. If you can't find a food you've eaten on the list, check food labels or other standard calorie-counting guides. (See Resources, page 235, for our recommended online calorie-lookup sites.)

It's better to add up the calories as you go, rather than waiting until later; that way you'll have a running tally of what you've eaten. But if you don't have time to do the math each time, don't sweat it. Do the best you can, and add up the numbers at the end of the day.

Take five. Plan on spending at least 5 minutes after each meal to work on your diary. Even if you're busy and stressed out— and who isn't?—five minutes isn't likely to make or break your day. It's about as much time as you spend taking a bathroom break, and nearly as essential to your well-being.

What about those check-off boxes? The boxes at the bottom of each page of the Food Diary are designed to help you make sure you get a minimum amount of some key nutritious foods each day. Just ignore them for your first week, and focus on getting in the habit of just writing down what you eat. More about those boxes in Chapter 2.

Do I Have to Write *Everything* Down?

There's no denying that keeping a food diary takes time, especially in the beginning as you learn the ropes. But there's also no denying that it really works. Simply put, studies show that people who use food diaries tend to lose more weight and keep it off longer than those who don't. *Food diaries are so important, we consider them essential. You'll see why in just a day or two.*

If you're feeling overwhelmed at the idea of a food diary, you're probably someone who will benefit the most from this kind of approach. It might be the first time that you've stepped back and really paid attention to your daily eating behavior, and you might be amazed at what it shows you about yourself.

Keep in mind that like all habits, recording in your food diary will get easier over time, as it becomes instinctive. You'll notice you eat many of the same foods from day to day, so you won't have to look up their calories every time. (Your previous days' diary entries will serve as a handy reference for calorie counts too.) You'll quickly memorize the calorie counts in your staples—about 70 in half an English muffin, 140 if you eat the whole thing, 35 more if you spread on a pat of butter.

> **"** Honesty is the first chapter in the book of wisdom. **"**
>
> THOMAS JEFFERSON

TRACK YOUR WEIGHT: IT WORKS!

Just like a food diary, recording your weight regularly is a powerful motivating tool. It can give you valuable feedback on how your weight-loss efforts are paying off and what's not working. Moreover, keeping track of your scale readings over time might help prevent you from gaining weight, even when you're surrounded by food temptations.

A recent report from Cornell University researchers sheds light on how weight tracking works, even in the food-centric environment of a first semester at college. (First-semester weight gain is so common it even has a name; students routinely dread putting on the "Freshman 15" in their first year of school.) In two successive studies, groups of freshmen women were instructed to weigh themselves daily and to e-mail the results to research staffers, who tracked their weights on a timeline and e-mailed the results to the women weekly. At the same time, "control" groups did no daily weighing. Neither group received any instruction on weight loss.

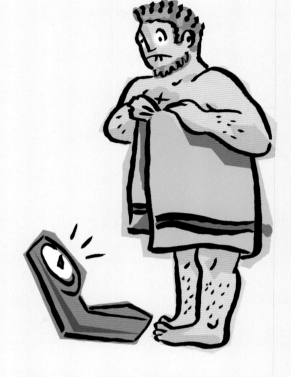

By the end of the semester, the women in the control groups had gained an average of about 4½ to 6 pounds. By contrast, weights of the women in the daily-weighing groups had remained essentially unchanged—suggesting that this regular "weight awareness check" was itself a tool for preventing weight gain. It's reasonable to project from these findings that regular weighing could also help prevent people from gaining back pounds after they've lost weight.

> **" Fat is not a moral problem. It's an oral problem. "**
>
> JANE THOMAS NOLAND, AUTHOR, *LAUGH IT OFF*

Since your weight can fluctuate greatly from day to day, it's not important to weigh yourself daily—but some people find it easier to remember that way. Weighing once weekly is fine too. Use the Weight Tracker Chart on page 239 to keep a record of your weight readings; it will give you a good long-term view of your weight loss. You'll see that the path to losing weight is never a straight line—some days you'll be up a pound or two, others down. But the long-term trend will show the pounds headed south.

However you choose to do your weighing, try to do it at the same time of the day, with the same amount of clothing (say, in your pajamas as soon as you wake up). Make sure your scale is calibrated (that it reads "0" when nobody's standing on it) and on a completely flat surface. Many people prefer a newer digital scale for easily getting a quick, precise reading rather than the old quivering pointer.

> **" Self-delusion is pulling in your stomach when you step on the scales. "**
>
> PAUL SWEENEY, HUMORIST

GET A GAME PLAN

In this chapter, you've set your long-term and starting weight-loss goals, and you're keeping your eyes on that prize. Good for you! But as we noted earlier, goals are easier to achieve when they're broken into smaller (and less intimidating) steps—a game plan.

So your long-term goal is "I want to lose weight." Think of smaller, more specific goals that will help you shed pounds, such as:

Eat fewer calories.

Burn more calories with exercise.

Now, continue to break each step down until you have a list of very specific changes you can make in order to accomplish your goal. How can you eat fewer calories? Here are a few examples:

SPECIFIC GOAL: Stop eating out so much

STRATEGY 1: Brown-bag lunch at work this week.

STRATEGY 2: Prepare big-batch meals on Sunday to have homemade dinners ready to warm up or finish throughout the week.

SPECIFIC GOAL: Cut back on snack foods

STRATEGY 1: Buy only one type of snack food (say, whole-wheat crackers).

STRATEGY 2: Keep snack foods in the back of the cupboard, out of sight.

Use the Game Plan Worksheet on page 28 to plan specific goals and strategies that work for you.

> **"** If you hang your swimsuit
> On the refrigerator door,
> The goodies inside
> Will be easier to ignore. **"**
>
> THE QUOTE GARDEN

ONLINE TRACKING TOOLS

You can use free software from the U.S. Department of Agriculture's "My Pyramid" program to create a food diary—with links to nutrition databases for nutrition/calorie information.

You can also use an online "MyPyramid Tracker" to record and track your weight for up to a year.

For details, check out **www.mypyramid.gov**.

GAME PLAN WORKSHEET

Write down three specific goals that will help you accomplish your big-picture goal of losing weight. Then, for each, come up with two game-plan strategies for getting there.

SPECIFIC GOAL:

_____

STRATEGY 1: _____

_____

STRATEGY 2: _____

_____

SPECIFIC GOAL:

_____

STRATEGY 1: _____

_____

STRATEGY 2: _____

_____

SPECIFIC GOAL:

_____

STRATEGY 1: _____

_____

STRATEGY 2: _____

_____

NOW YOU TRY IT: TRACK YOURSELF

After taking the "test run" earlier in this chapter, you're ready to start your food diary. Print out a week's worth of pages and start building your personal history. Put your calorie goal at the top of each page, and do your best to come close to it each day—but don't beat yourself up if you're off by a fair margin at first. Seeing the eating habits you have now will give you some good clues about how you can make changes later. Your focus should be on recording everything and anything. If you're using the Mix & Match Menus (see page 86) to plan some or all of your meals, we've already done the calorie counting for you.

As you make your entries this week, use the "Notes" section to record thoughts and situations that influence your eating patterns. All that information will be helpful as you work on adapting healthier habits and behaviors. Keep the following questions in mind:

Where do you do most of your eating?

_____

_____

_____

When are you most likely to overeat?

_____

_____

_____

When and where is it easiest for you NOT to eat?

_____

_____

_____

What other people have positive or negative effects on your eating?

_____

_____

_____

What kinds of foods contribute most to your total calorie intake?

_____

_____

_____

CHAPTER 2

BECOME FOOD WISE

THE POWER OF KNOWING WHAT YOU ARE PUTTING IN YOUR BODY

Eating well is so much more than counting calories. If it were that simple, you could meet, easily and without a second thought, a 1,200-calorie daily goal just by sipping three fast-food chocolate milkshakes. Think of how you could amaze friends by saying you were on the Mocha Shake Diet.

Unfortunately, I can say with complete confidence that it wouldn't leave you feeling satisfied for long. Within a relatively few "meals" you would be sick of cheap chocolate flavoring and faux creaminess. You would be craving something, anything, else. (You've just discovered the secret of those "eat only [insert specific food here]" diets: we humans find having the same thing over and over again is so boring, it kills our appetite—at least for the particular food or foods that make up the diet. We eat less, lose some weight, then can stand it no longer and go back to eating a variety of foods.)

When you think about the diets you've tried and left in the dust, most have likely made very rigid recommendations about eating. Many vilify one type of food, or even make a whole category of foods off limits (carbs, anyone?), while ascribing almost magical properties to another food (say, protein, brown rice or grapefruit). Others insist you combine foods in certain ways or only eat them at certain times.

Surprise: I acknowledge that many such diets can work. Limiting food choices, especially in an environment where we're bombarded with a huge selection of food offerings every day, is a powerful strategy. But when it comes to finding a way to live the rest of your life, turning yourself into someone with peculiar food habits is hard to sustain for long. Having to defend your weird food issues to family and friends, day in and day out, can wear you down—just as effectively as the food limitations get more and more confining. If you've tried any of the popular food-restricting diets, did you lose weight on that plan? And you stuck with the diet for how long? And you gained the weight back when? I rest my case.

> **"**The alimentary canal is thirty-two feet long. You control only the first three inches of it. Control it well.**"**
>
> KIN HUBBARD, HUMORIST

STEP 4: EAT MINDFULLY

You've heard it before: Healthy eating means getting a variety of foods in moderate portions. It means not making any food forbidden, but at the same time not going overboard on those rich foods that were once special-occasion indulgences and now surround us almost daily. It means means moving to Step 3 of your weight loss journey, becoming a person who eats mindfully. That's quite different from a diet zealot who shuns what everyone else is eating. In the previous chapter, you started getting a handle on calorie awareness and how to set your daily caloric goals. Now you'll begin to develop and hone your skills at choosing foods wisely and portioning them in sensible amounts. You'll work on identifying foods that might trigger you to overeat, as well as those that can help you stay focused on your healthy-eating strategies. You'll even pick up a few new ways to eat. Most important, you'll find a way to lose weight that lets you be true to yourself—that lets you be you!

WHAT'S A HEALTHY WAY TO EAT?

For an overall snapshot of what a balanced diet looks like, the U.S. Department of Agriculture (USDA)'s "MyPyramid" recommendations are a pretty good start. They divide foods into recognizable groupings, provide standard serving sizes for foods within each group, and suggest a range of servings you can aim to eat daily.

The food groups are fairly straightforward: grains and other starches, vegetables, fruits, milk products, meats and beans, oils and "discretionary calories," or extras. The whole USDA Pyramid is now meant to be viewed online (www.mypyramid.gov) and is a highly visual depiction of one way to approach healthful eating.

However, unless you read a lot of fine print in the MyPyramid guidelines, you might not get a clear sense of what it all means if you're trying to limit calories too.

Just to keep things simple, let's think of your calorie goal as a daily budget to work with. And, while you can spend your budget any way you want, it makes sense to get the best value for your "money" by choosing the widest selection of items—that is, eating from all the food groups. Let's take a closer look at the kinds of foods you can choose from each day and—importantly—how much you might choose from each major group.

> **"To change your life: start immediately; do it flamboyantly; no exceptions."**
>
> WILLIAM JAMES

GRAINS AND STARCHY VEGETABLES

One serving or "ounce equivalent" =
- **1 slice bread**
- **½ English muffin**
- **½ medium (2-ounce) bagel**
- **1 ounce cold cereal (varies widely, from ¼ cup granola to 2 cups puffed rice)**
- **½ cup cooked rice, pasta, winter squash, corn *or* hot cereal**
- **½ medium (3-4-ounce) potato or sweet potato**

In this category are foods rich in carbohydrates—the body's main fuel supply—so we need a fair amount daily (despite what the low-carb/no-carb gurus say). The key is to keep portions moderate and skew strongly to the better choices. This can be tough for weight-conscious people: since white pasta, white potatoes and white bread are cheap and abundant, they're often served in gargantuan portions.

> I'm not much of a junk-food junkie—I'm interested in eating healthy, and I eat good foods. My problem is I just eat too much.
> —**Jan**, 47 (58 pounds lost)

Within this group, trade up to whole-grain versions—whole-grain bread, pasta, brown rice—as often as you can. Similarly, choose potatoes with skin on for more fiber and nutrients. You'll feel fuller longer, since whole grains and fiber take longer to digest. There is also the significant bonus of getting a healthy boost of vitamins, minerals and fiber as well as antioxidants and other so-called "phytonutrients." While the government guidelines urge you to "make half of your grains whole," we say aim for making most, if not all, of your grains whole. The variety and eating quality of whole-grain products have grown by leaps and bounds in recent years, making it easy to relegate the refined, "white" versions to special uses and occasions. (*See "The Glycemic Index," page 38.*)

NONSTARCHY VEGETABLES

One serving =
  1 cup leafy vegetables
  ½ cup cooked vegetables
  ¾ cup vegetable juice

Load up your plate! Most of these nonstarchy vegetables are practically calorie-free, but packed with antioxidants, vitamins, minerals and other key nutrients. There's probably no better nutrition bargain in the supermarket. You've heard the "5 a day" urging to eat at least five servings of vegetables (and fruits) daily. Most of us don't even come close, but more is even better. Studies suggest that a vegetable-rich diet with as many as 10 servings a day may help prevent cancer, heart disease, stroke and high blood pressure, and it's also a smart weight-loss strategy. Consider "5 a day" a minimum. Just doing that will put you well on the way toward eating a lower-calorie diet (*see "Eat More, Get Less,"* *page 36*).

Try to vary your vegetables, making sure you get a variety of colors—vegetable pigments are especially good sources of phytonutrients. Try dark green kale and broccoli, orange-yellow carrots, deep-red beets. Getting enough isn't as tall an order as it sounds, since a serving is a mere ½ cup for most vegetables. Have a good handful of baby carrots and you've already had two servings.

> *Make it a habit to eat a piece of fruit in the morning, and at least a cup of vegetables at lunch and dinner. That's "5 a day" without breaking a sweat.*

> **"** This cabbage, these carrots, these potatoes, these onions…will soon become me. Such a tasty fact! **"**
>
> MICHAEL GAROFALO,
> POET & GARDENER

FRUITS

One serving =
  1 medium fruit
  ½ cup chopped *or* canned fruit
  ¾ cup fruit juice

Fruit is a luscious way to satisfy a craving for sweetness and pleasure, without adding a lot of calories. Get in the habit of eating at least 2 pieces of fresh fruit daily; a small piece (say, a small apple) or ½ cup chopped fruit constitutes one serving. Like vegetables, fruits are great sources of vitamins (especially vitamin C), minerals and phytonutrients, such as the antioxidants lycopene (in reddish pigments in watermelon) and beta carotene (in yellow-orange fruits like mango and peaches). And, when you eat them whole rather than drinking their juice, you have the heart-healthy, satiety-enhancing effects of their fiber too. You can enjoy dried fruit, too, but it packs significantly more calories, so stick with a ¼-cup serving.

> *Try not to drink your fruits too often—their calories will go down with you hardly noticing. Enjoy the whole fruit instead—it's more satisfying.*

MILK AND OTHER CALCIUM-RICH FOODS

One serving =
> **1 cup milk, soymilk, yogurt *or* low-fat cottage cheese**
> **1½ ounces cheese (preferably reduced-fat)**

No matter how many calories you're budgeting, you'll want to include calcium-rich foods like low-fat or fat-free milk, cottage cheese or yogurt each day, to help keep your bones strong. Soy-based versions of these are fine, too, as long as they're fortified with vitamin D and calcium—two bone-building nutrients milk supplies abundantly. Dairy foods are also decent sources of protein, which helps add staying power to meals. Just be sure to choose low-fat or fat-free versions, or the calories quickly add up. Likewise, use full-fat cheese sparingly; it's high in calories and saturated fat. Choose one with strong flavor so a little goes a long way.

If you don't eat or can't tolerate dairy foods or fortified soymilk products, you can get your calcium from nondairy sources like dark green leafy vegetables and calcium-fortified products like orange juice and cereals—but they lack the protein benefits of milk and may not contain vitamin D, so you'll need to get those nutrients elsewhere.

PROTEIN GROUP

One serving or "ounce equivalent" =
> **1 ounce cooked meat, poultry *or* fish**
> **¼ cup cooked beans or legumes**
> **1 large egg**
> **2 tablespoons peanut butter**
> **1 ounce (small handful) nuts**
> **3 ounces tofu**

This grouping contains foods rich in protein, including meats, poultry, seafood, eggs, tofu, beans, nuts and legumes. They supply the amino acids needed to build the tissues of the body—most

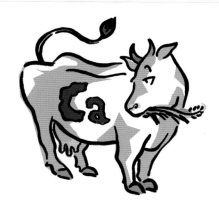

Is Milk a Magic Bullet for Losing Weight?

Not long ago, a few intriguing studies (funded by the dairy industry) suggested that weight-loss diets that included three to four daily servings of milk or other dairy foods were more effective in both shedding pounds and burning fat than conventional diets. But when we set out to repeat those findings at our research center at the University of Vermont, our results were, frankly, disappointing.

In our study, 54 overweight, middle-aged men and women followed a weight-loss plan much like the one you're holding in your hands now, with plenty of exercise and behavior-modification tips. We divided them into two equal groups, and prescribed an eating plan that included the same amount of calories for both. The only difference was that one eating plan provided three or four servings of low-fat dairy foods daily, while the other served up just one daily dairy serving. After six months, the high-dairy group had lost about 22 pounds, on average; the low-dairy group, about 20½ pounds; statistically, that's a dead heat with the difference so small it could be due simply to chance. What does this tell us? Dairy foods are probably not a magic bullet for increasing weight loss—but that doesn't mean they're not important. There's no better source of bone-building calcium, after all. And the good news is that you can lose weight without having to cut your dairy intake (as some people tend to do), as long as you watch the fat content. Just don't expect any weight-loss magic from milk.

famously, muscle tissue. Note, too, that a little protein added to a meal can really make it more satisfying, so if you're having trouble with between-meal hunger pangs, try to incorporate a portion of protein into each meal: a tablespoon of chopped almonds on your morning oatmeal, some shredded chicken breast on your lunch salad, and a cup of bean soup at dinner, for example.

Fat is very energy-dense, so lean protein sources are your best bet to keep calories low. Trim skin from poultry and choose lean meat cuts like the various types of loin and sirloin. The only exception to the "lean is better" rule is with fatty fish like salmon, tuna and sardines, because the fat they contain is rich in heart-healthy omega-3 fatty acids. That's why the American Heart Association recommends getting two 3-ounce servings of fish per week—"preferably fatty fish." Also, try to include some vegetable sources of protein in your diet regularly, to get a good dose of fiber along with your protein. Beans and soyfoods like tofu, tempeh and meat substitutes are terrific. Nuts are excellent protein sources, but quite high in calories, so pay attention to the relatively small size of a single serving: just 2 tablespoons peanut butter, and a small handful of nuts (14 almonds), for example.

> **" You've got bad eating habits if you use a grocery cart in 7-Eleven, okay? "**
>
> DENNIS MILLER, COMEDIAN

OILS
One serving =
- **1 teaspoon oil**
- **1 tablespoon vinaigrette dressing**
- **2 teaspoons creamy salad dressing**
- **5 large olives**
- **⅛ avocado**

The days of single-minded fat phobia are officially over. We now recognize that olive, canola, sunflower, safflower, corn, soybean and nut oils are important sources of fat-soluble vitamins, and they help make foods taste delicious, no small contribution (*see "But Isn't Fat Fattening?" page 36*). And, like all fats that are liquid at room temperature, they're unsaturated fats, which can protect the heart by helping prevent cholesterol buildup in

Servings vs. portions

Note that a "serving" and a "portion" are often used interchangeably, but they're not the same thing. A serving is a standard unit of measure, for example, one egg or half a hamburger bun—as established by nutritionists and published in government documents. But a portion refers to how much food we actually eat—two eggs scrambled, perhaps, or the whole burger bun. So, while technically ½ cup of spaghetti is "one serving," few of us would actually consider that a "portion." (Some might consider it the first forkful.) A spaghetti *portion* of 1 cup, or even 1 ½ cups, is more realistic. But if that's what you're eating, know that you've eaten two or three servings of grain-based foods when you dig into that bowl of pasta. (*See Portions Visualized, page 40.*)

arteries. Especially heart-healthy are sources rich in so-called "monounsaturated" fats, including olive, canola and "high-oleic" sunflower or safflower oil, as well as avocados and olives.

Note that fats like butter, lard, shortening and cream don't fit into this category—these "solid fats" (thus named because they're solid at room temperature) contain too much saturated fat to qualify as a daily staple. Instead, they're counted as "discretionary" calories (see below) to use as occasional luxuries.

DISCRETIONARY CALORIES

Think of this category as a "slush fund"—some additional calories to use for those little extras that don't fit into the other food categories. Use these calories for a glass of wine, a sweet treat, a fast-food goody, or foods whose saturated fat or calorie content keeps them off of the rest of the healthy pyramid—like bacon, butter, cream, full-fat cheese and cream cheese. Once you've met your daily goals from the other food groups, there often aren't a lot of extra calories to play around with, so choose your discretionary calories—well, with discretion.

You can "bank" discretionary calories if you like, to use for an upcoming splurge—say, a birthday party or a restaurant night out. Just keep track of unused calories in your diary, and try to use them up within a week.

NOW YOU TRY IT: SERVINGS QUIZ

How many food group servings does this meal reflect?

Entree:	1½ cups penne pasta with ½ cup tomato sauce
Salad:	2 cups lettuce, ½ cup chopped tomatoes, ½ cup cooked chickpeas, 1 tablespoon balsamic vinaigrette dressing
Side Dish:	1 cup fresh fruit salad
Beverage:	8-ounce glass of skim milk

Grains and Starchy Vegetables _____
Nonstarchy Vegetables _____
Fruit _____
Milk/Calcium-Rich Foods _____
Protein Group _____
Oils _____

Answers to "NOW YOU TRY IT"

Grains and Starchy Vegetables: 3
Nonstarchy Vegetables: 4
Fruit: 2
Milk/Calcium-Rich Foods: 1
Protein Group: 2
Oils: 1

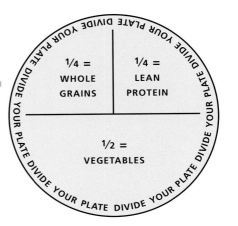

Divide Your Plate

Confused by servings and portions? Here's a quick way to ensure you're eating a good balance of foods. Imagine a plate and divide it in half. Fill one half with vegetables. Divide the other half into two equal portions (quarters), and fill one with a lean protein. Fill the other quarter with a whole-grain food or starchy vegetable. Try to make most of your meals look like this, and you're well on your way to good nutrition.

"BUT ISN'T FAT FATTENING?"

Many people entering weight-loss programs ask, "Shouldn't I be cutting out all fat?" When you're trying to lose weight, it's easy to cast fat in the role of the nutritional bad guy. After all, fat contains more than twice as many calories (9 per gram) as the other key food components we eat, protein and carbohydrates (both 4 calories per gram). So when you cut fat from foods, you get more bang for your calorie-cutting buck. Why not just slash fat from the menu?

From a weight-loss standpoint, it makes sense to be moderate with fat—but that includes not cutting it out immoderately, either. Adding a bit of fat to a food makes the digestion process take a little longer, prolonging fullness and helping you feel satisfied. It also aids the absorption of fat-soluble vitamins like A, D and E. But perhaps most importantly, fat helps make food pleasurable. It contributes and carries flavors and, as a cooking medium, adds all kinds of textures to foods, from creaminess to crispy crunch. And let's face it, without a little salad dressing or a bit of a flavorful sauce, many vegetables wouldn't get eaten, no matter how "good for us" they are.

Pleasure is a key component of designing a lifetime eating strategy. If you aren't enjoying what you eat, you won't eat it for long, so don't defat your food to the point of tastelessness. (Just think of all those ghastly "fat-free" foods that cropped up on grocery shelves during the fat-scare decade of the 1990s. Most are history now.) If you're aware of the serving sizes for fats and use a light touch when adding them to foods—for example, spreading no more than a measured teaspoon of mayonnaise on your sandwich—you'll enjoy it in moderation and soon won't miss the usual overload that gives fat a bad name.

EAT MORE, GET LESS

Start edging up the amount of produce in your daily diet and chances are good that you'll eat fewer calories without even noticing. A recent look at the massive Continuing Survey of Food Intakes by Individuals (CSFII)—the government's chief survey of American eating habits—found that men and women with the highest average vegetable and fruit intakes (more than 4½ cups daily) tended to have the lowest rates of obesity. And, even though they ate a greater amount of food, their actual calorie intake was lower, since their produce-rich diets were in effect "watered down" with low-calorie fruits and vegetables.

The Check-Off Boxes: Turbo-Charge Your Food Diary

By now you're probably getting more comfortable with keeping a daily food diary and tracking your daily calorie intake. That's terrific, since limiting your calories is the critical pathway to losing weight successfully. But perhaps you'd like a little more guidance on how to structure your daily meals within those calorie limits.

That's why we've included an optional "Key Foods Checklist" at the bottom of each EATINGWELL Food Diary page. The list includes 5 categories of foods we consider critical to any healthy eating pattern, with a series of boxes following each. Each box represents one serving from that food group, and the number of boxes gives you a minimum number of servings to aim for daily, no matter what your calorie range. (To keep things simple, we didn't include foods you shouldn't have trouble getting enough of, like oils, refined grains and sweets.) If you've filled all the boxes by the end of the day, you'll have eaten wisely and well, with calories left over to use as you like.

Here's how the Key Foods Checklist stacks up:

Nonstarchy Vegetables: 5 - 10 servings

Fruits: 2 servings

Whole Grains: 3 servings

Protein Group: 5-6 (1-ounce) servings

Calcium-Rich Foods: 2 daily servings

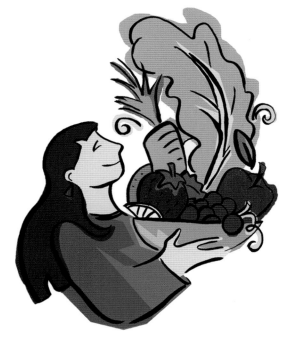

The "Key Foods Checklist" boxes in the EatingWell Food Diary are strictly optional. But do give them a try occasionally. It's a great way to check in and see how you're doing nutritionally.

THE GLYCEMIC INDEX

I'm often asked what I think about the Glycemic Index—a system of ranking foods by how quickly the carbohydrates in them are digested. I usually respond that it's a terrific principle—but only if you don't get too hung up on the numbers. Technically, knowing where the foods you eat fall on the glycemic scale can help point you toward making healthier food choices and better controlling your hunger, but it's important to understand the limitation of this approach too.

How does the glycemic index work? It starts with glucose—a form of sugar that's used to fuel the body's cells. Our bodies break down just about everything we eat (especially carbohydrates) into glucose, which is released directly into the bloodstream where it can travel to all the places it's needed. But to get into cells, glucose needs an escort: insulin, a hormone made in the pancreas. Think of insulin as the "key" that unlocks the door to your cells, allowing glucose to get inside.

When you eat something and produce glucose, your pancreas kicks into action, releasing just enough insulin to usher the available glucose into cells. This causes blood-glucose (blood-sugar) levels to drop, and after that, a decrease in insulin levels. Eat again, and the cycle starts all over: glucose rises, insulin rises; glucose drops, insulin drops. That's a pretty sophisticated system of checks and balances.

Problems arise when we eat foods that break down very quickly into glucose: refined carbohydrates like sweets, soft drinks, white breads, white potatoes and such. Eating these foods triggers a fast rise in blood sugar, and with it, a flood of insulin—a so-called "insulin peak"—and very soon, blood-glucose levels drop precipitously. That can cause you to feel hungry pretty quickly—sometimes even hungrier than before you started eating! That's why munching a handful of jelly beans (or guzzling a can of regular soda) doesn't put a dent in your hunger when you're ravenous.

By contrast, if you choose carbohydrate foods that are more slowly digested—including whole grains, vegetables and beans and other legumes—the subsequent blood-sugar rise is much gentler and slower, and so is the insulin release that follows. You get a lower insulin peak, and thus your blood-sugar levels fall more slowly; you won't feel hungry again for a while. That's why a morning bowl of (whole-grain) oatmeal sticks with you longer, leaving you less hungry at lunchtime.

How to tell which foods are quick-digesting or slow burners? That's where the glycemic index (GI) comes in. It ranks carbohydrate foods based on how much a food containing 50 grams of carbohydrate raises blood-glucose levels after eating. This value is compared with the response to a reference food given a GI of 100—usually pure glucose or white bread. A food with a GI less than 55 is considered low, while anything more than 70 is high. You might also use a similar system of ranking carbohydrate foods—the glycemic load (GL), which considers both a food's GI and how much carbohydrate the food contains in a standard portion. With both systems, lower is better.

Here's where I part ways with GI/GL number crunching: Most of our meals don't consist of just one food item—we eat combinations of different foods, all of which can influence the glycemic value of the meal in different ways. Just adding a pat of butter to a potato will lower its glycemic value significantly, for example, since fat molecules take longer for the body to digest. Sprinkling cheese on a bowl of pasta will have the same effect. So while the GI and

> **All people are made alike. They are made of bone, flesh and dinners. Only the dinners are different.**
>
> GERTRUDE LOUISE CHENEY, CHILD POET

GL are one tool for pointing you toward healthier eating and curbing hunger, they're not the last word.

Studies show that people who eat foods with lower glycemic indices tend to be leaner, and have lower risk of developing diabetes. But can following a program of eating low-glycemic index foods help you lose weight? While some clinical studies suggest it can help, others show no effect, so clearly the answers aren't in yet.

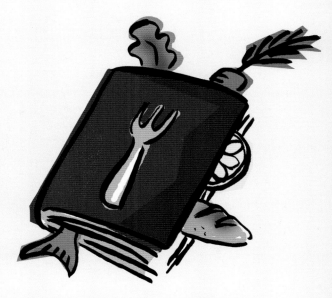

But for the most part, glycemic rankings make intuitive sense, so you don't have to fuss too much with the numbers. Most of the so-called "healthy" foods you probably try to eat more of are low on the glycemic scale—like vegetables, whole grains, beans and other high-fiber foods. And the foods with higher glycemic values, like refined grains and sweets, are probably ones you've aimed to avoid anyway. Here are good rules of thumb for lowering the glycemic values of what you eat daily:

Don't be refined. Watch your intake of foods and products made with refined grains, such as white bread or white rice, crackers, potatoes and pasta, and choose unrefined (whole-grain) versions of these foods whenever possible. It's getting a lot easier—just look at how many whole-grain pastas you can find these days. Try mixing them half and half with their refined counterparts at first, then gradually phase in more whole grains as you become used to them.

Fiber up. Experts recommend that we get 25-30 grams of fiber daily, but most of us barely meet the halfway mark. Aim for that goal, and you'll also be lowering the glycemic values of your meals by making them move more slowly through your digestive system. Try reading labels and selecting packaged foods with highest fiber content; leave the peels on vegetables and fruits when they're edible. Make your default breakfast a high-fiber cereal; shop around to find a brand you like that provides at least 8 grams of fiber per serving. Try to eat beans, lentils, split peas or other legumes at least three times a week; snack on fiber-rich foods like popcorn, high-fiber crispbreads, and nuts and dried fruits in moderation.

Pair with protein. Whenever you're eating a carbohydrate-based meal or snack, make sure there's at least a little protein in the mix—some chicken strips in your pasta bowl or a light smear of peanut butter on your English muffin, for example. Protein takes longer to digest than carbohydrates, so you'll have a more gradual rise and fall of blood sugar—and you'll feel fuller longer too.

Drizzle with a little oil. Fats, like proteins, are broken down into large particles that take a longer time for the body to digest—so adding a little fat to a carbohydrate-rich meal can lessen its glycemic impact considerably. Drizzle bread with a little olive oil; toss carrots with a bit of tasty dressing. Keep in mind, though, that fat calories add up more than twice as fast as those of protein or carbohydrate—so drizzle judiciously.

Double-check. Curious about the GI/GL score of your favorite foods? It might be useful—and sometimes eye-opening—to know. So you don't get bogged down in details, just focus on foods you eat most often, such as breakfast cereal or particular fruits. Check www.eatingwell.com/diet for a link to an international table of glycemic index and glycemic load values, compiled by researchers at the University of Sydney, Australia, and published in the *American Journal of Clinical Nutrition*.

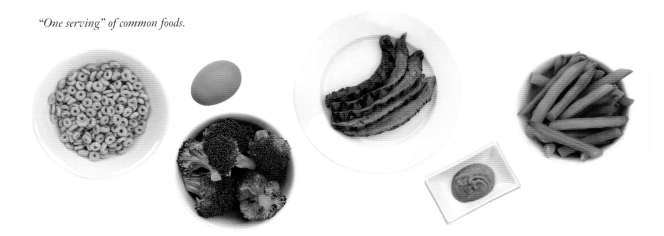

"One serving" of common foods.

PORTIONS VISUALIZED: A GRAPHIC REALITY CHECK

As a society, we're eating more calories than ever, and a leading culprit is how often we eat prepared foods away from home. And, whether they come from a restaurant, takeout or vending machine, the portions we're being served are often larger than life. According to one study, most marketplace food portions can be two to eight times larger than standard portion sizes. While the USDA considers a "medium" bagel to be about 2 ounces, the behemoths you find at a bagel store today can weigh in at 5 ounces—equivalent to 5 slices of bread! A jumbo baked potato at a restaurant might equal 6 to 8 slices of bread. Pretty hefty for what most people consider a side dish.

With the advent of megasized meals, jumbo muffins and extra-big drink cups, many of us have lost touch with what proper portions look like. We've gotten so used to seeing these oversized helpings that we think they're normal—and that anything else looks skimpy. The problem just deepens as restaurant portion sizes creep into the plate-filling habits of home cooks.

Part of learning how to eat better, then, is to retrain your brain to recognize—and embrace—more realistic portion sizes.

With time, portion-size awareness tends to fade—and the amounts we serve ourselves tend to creep up. Even if you feel you've mastered the art of proper portioning, plan on rechecking yourself regularly with standard measuring utensils.

If you're reaching for seconds every time you sit down to dinner, you're not likely to lose much weight. Likewise, if you clean your plate at restaurants, you're almost guaranteed to be overeating.

THINK SMALL

So we're being served larger helpings; everyone around us seems to be eating larger amounts. How does a mindful eater avoid following the crowd and downing three or four portions at a time? Here are some tried-and-true techniques from successful weight "losers":

Use smaller serving pieces: A 7-inch plate, about the size of a "salad" plate or children's-size plate is ideal for your main meal. Choose a 1-cup dessert or cereal bowl instead of a soup bowl, a 6-ounce wineglass rather than a goblet. By the way, research shows you'll think you have more to drink when you pour it into a tall, thin glass rather than a short, wide one (save those big glasses for calorie-free water and sparkling water).

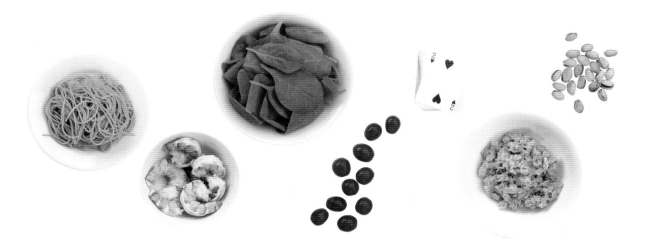

Use the chart below to help you visualize the correct portion sizes of the foods you eat most often. Make an effort to measure out portions you serve yourself and you'll soon be able to "eyeball" them accurately.

MEASURING WITH YOUR EYES	
1 teaspoon	About the size of your fingertip (tip to middle joint); fits into the screwcap of a water bottle
1 tablespoon	About the size of your thumb tip (tip to middle joint)
½ cup	A fruit or vegetable that fits into the palm of your hand—about the size of a tennis ball
¼ cup	A golf ball
1 ounce nuts	Fits into the cupped palm of a child's hand
1 cup cereal	About the size of a woman's fist or a baseball
1 medium bagel	A hockey puck
1 ounce cheese	About the size of 2 dominoes or 4 dice
3 ounces meat	About the size of a deck of cards or a cassette audiotape
1 medium potato	About the size of a computer mouse

Train your eye: In your own kitchen, have a little session in which you measure out an accurate portion of the foods you eat regularly—say, cereal, soup, pasta, pretzels—into one type of bowl, so you'll imprint a visual memory of how they look and just how they fill the bowl. Use that bowl every time you eat that food. (Extra credit: Use a permanent marker to write the amount of food the bowl holds on the bottom of the bowl. Then you'll always know what you're getting.)

Ask for an extra salad plate: In a restaurant, get a smaller side plate or hold on to the bread plate, if it's large enough, and transfer the proper-size portions of your food onto it when you're served your entree. Ask the waiter to take away and wrap up the rest. (*For more restaurant tips, see Chapter 4.*)

Buy single-serving packages: Do this for all tempting foods—snack-size cookie or chip bags, pudding cups, fun-size candy bars. Or divide a larger package into single portions and put them in individual small plastic bags.

Read labels: Make sure you're eating a single portion of packaged foods. If your bag of pretzels has 2 servings, take out half and put the rest away for tomorrow's snack.

Cook up calorie-rich foods in pre-portioned sizes: Divide casseroles into ramekins, bake mini cupcakes rather than cakes, make meatloaf in muffin cups.

> **"**We never repent of having eaten too little.**"**
> THOMAS JEFFERSON

FOOD SHOPPING 101

Your goal is to stock up on healthy foods and only buy what you truly need. But stop and remember that your supermarket's goal, of course, is to get you to buy as much as possible. Between the enticing free samples (why are they always serving pizza?) and the display of potato chips at the end of the aisle where you're bound to see them, it might seem as if the place is booby-trapped. Here are a few tips to keep you on course.

Have a plan. Spend 15 minutes at the beginning of the week to plan out healthy meals for the rest of the week, and make a list of the ingredients you'll need. Keep a running list and post it on the fridge so you can write down what you need as you remember it.

Never shop without a list in hand. You'll be less likely to be tempted by impulse buys. Use the "EATINGWELL Pantry" on page 244 to stock your cupboards, refrigerator and freezer, and visit www.eatingwell.com/diet for more ideas and tips.

Never shop hungry. Go to the store after you've had a meal, so an empty stomach won't tempt you to buy more. If you can't, have an apple or other healthy snack before you go in.

Shop the periphery. Generally, you'll find whole foods (fresh produce, dairy) along the sides and back of the store. Packaged goods, including tempting snacks, are usually concentrated in the center aisles.

Read labels. Take the time to compare packaged foods to find a brand you like with a nutritional profile that works with your health goals. Focus on just one or two food categories on each shopping trip, so you won't be

How to Eat

Your eating patterns—such as the timing between mouthfuls and the order in which you eat the food on your plate—can have a real impact on how many calories you consume in a day. Modifying these little details to work in your favor can be a help when you're trying to lose weight. Here are some simple tactics that can help you cut calories without changing *what* you eat.

Designate one eating place. Restrict all your eating to one location, such as the kitchen or dining room table. It should be comfortable, but not filled with distractions like television, reading material or computer screens. By luring your focus away from your food, they can make you eat more. You may also start pairing or associating eating with an activity, like watching television. It's bad enough that television commercials tempt us with high-calorie food advertisements, but if just turning the box on makes you start thinking "eat now," it's that much harder to stay on track.

Don't come to the table ravenous. Your hunger could easily drive you to go overboard, and you'll wolf down more food than you need before you know it. Try not to let more than five hours elapse between meals, and never skip a meal.

Eat only on plates and bowls. This helps reinforce that you're eating a meal, and that it has a beginning and an end.

overwhelmed with information. Try comparing whole-grain crackers on one trip, jars of pasta sauce on another, for example.

A CLOSER LOOK AT THE LABEL

By law, packaged foods sold in the U.S. have a standardized Nutrition Facts Panel, which gives a lot of helpful information for those trying to make a lower-calorie or more healthful choice—if you focus on these key areas.

Serving size: To make comparing foods easier, similar foods must have similar serving sizes—but "one serving" might not be what you consume in one sitting. Always check serving size and adjust accordingly; if a serving size is 15 potato chips and you eat 30, double the rest of the nutrition information you're counting too.

Calories: Again, these just reflect a count for a single serving, and you'll need to adjust if you eat more or less. The "calories from fat" column can give you an idea of the extent to which fat influences the calorie content.

Key nutrients: Nutrient labels list amounts of those nutrients that supply energy (e.g., calories): carbohydrates, protein and fats, with some categories broken down further. The ones worth noting are:

Saturated Fat: As low as possible (under 3 grams/serving).

Trans Fat: Should be "0."

Cholesterol: As low as possible (daily goal: 300 mg or less).

Sodium: As low as possible (Dietary Guidelines recommendation: 2,300 mg/day or less).

Dietary Fiber: As high as possible (daily goal is 25 grams or more).

Sugars: Interesting but not always useful, since labels don't discriminate between naturally occurring sugars (such as in milk or fruit) and added sugars.

Vitamins and minerals: Vitamins A and C, calcium and iron are required to be listed on labels since consuming enough of these nutrients can improve your health and reduce your risk of some diseases. They're shown in the form of Daily Values.

Percent Daily Values (DVs). These are reference amounts set by the Food and Drug Administration (FDA). You can use Daily Values to help you track how much of your nutrient needs that food fills. But take

Don't take serving bowls to the table. Keep the food on the kitchen counter and just carry your plate to the table. Leaving the serving bowls on the table makes it way too easy to take seconds.

Fill up on fiber first. Loading up on high-fiber foods like vegetables helps you feel full and can prevent you from overdoing on higher-calorie fare later. Start the meal with salad, a broth-based vegetable soup, some fresh fruit or a vegetable side dish.

Slow down. It takes about 20 minutes for "I'm full" signals to reach your brain. If you've inhaled an entire meal in 13 minutes, those satiety messages haven't had enough time to signal that you've eaten four portions. So put down the fork or spoon between each bite. (Some people find that eating with smaller utensils—like a teaspoon instead of a soup spoon, or chopsticks—helps them stay on a slower pace.) Chat with your dining companions—or if you're alone, take some relaxing breaths.

Listen to your body. Think of your hunger on a scale of 1 to 5, with 1 being "ravenous" and 5 being "stuffed." Stop eating when you've reached about 3 or 4 on the scale—that point where you're comfortably satisfied, but you could still eat a bit more.

AISLE BY AISLE:
A SUPERMARKET BUYING GUIDE

Produce: Let yourself be seduced here; fill your cart with plenty of colorful produce. Aim to try something new each week—an exotic fruit, or a vegetable you've never seen before—even if it costs a little more. You might discover a new healthy passion. Likewise, prewashed, ready-to-eat produce like salad mixes, baby carrots and broccoli/cauliflower florets may seem a splurge, but not if they get you to grab them instead of chips when you're craving a snack. (Admit it: would you pinch pennies so vigorously in the snack-food aisle?)

Poultry/Fish/Meat: If convenience is all-important, go for skinless poultry cuts and boneless for quickest cooking. You'll save some calories and fat by choosing white meat over dark, too—but don't sweat the difference if you're planning to broil or grill; most of the fat will drip off anyway. For ground chicken or turkey, make sure you're getting lean breast meat without skin added (read the label).

In the fish department, you can opt for white-fleshed fish for fewest calories, but don't forget fatty fish like salmon or tuna, which contain omega-3 fatty acids that dramatically lower your risk of heart attack and stroke

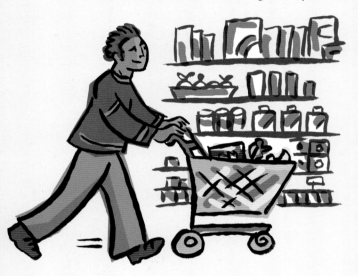

if eaten regularly; just choose a moderate portion to keep a lid on calories. Ask which fish is freshest (or check the Date Packed if it's precut) and reject anything that looks suspect or smells fishy (if it's wrapped in plastic, fillets should be firm to the touch, with no liquid in the package—a sign of improper thawing). Frozen fish is just fine—and sometimes it's the "freshest" choice. Just be sure to thaw it properly: overnight in the refrigerator.

Many successful weight-loss veterans make red meat a special-occasion rather than daily purchase, since it's higher in saturated fat. Look for cuts with "loin" or "round" in the title, and select well-trimmed cuts with the least visible fat. Choose ground beef labeled "90% lean" or higher.

Dairy: Seek out dairy products that get 30 percent or fewer calories from fat. When choosing milk, opt for "skim," "fat-free/nonfat" or "1 percent." (Avoid the misleadingly labeled "reduced-fat" 2 percent milk; about 36 percent of its calories come from fat.) However, "low-fat" (1 percent) or "nonfat" yogurts, cottage cheese and sour cream are all worth trying. If you're buying soy or rice "milk," check the label to make sure it's fortified with calcium and vitamin D—and to make sure you're aware of any added sugars.

Don't be afraid to experiment with lower-fat cheeses like part-skim mozzarella or Jarlsberg or reduced-fat Cheddars; they've improved greatly in recent years. (You can always blend them with a little full-fat cheese to boost flavor and texture.) Buy full-fat cheeses with strong flavors, like feta, blue, Parmesan or aged Cheddar—and count on just a little bit going a long way. If you buy butter, plan on using it sparingly—slice off a half-stick and store the rest in the freezer. Or if you prefer a buttery spread, read labels to find one that's free of heart-threatening trans fats. Don't forget the eggs—at 75 calories apiece, they're a diet-friendly protein source (and, contrary to popular belief, don't raise most people's blood cholesterol noticeably, since their saturated-fat content is fairly low). Fat-free egg substitutes (mostly consisting of egg white) are an even better calorie bargain; they're only about 30 calories per ¼-cup serving, though you might find them a bit bland compared to whole eggs.

Freezer: Stock up on plain frozen vegetables (shun the ones with sauce or butter) so that you've always got some veggies on hand. Most are frozen right after picking to preserve nutrients and flavor, so you don't have to feel you're compromising. You might also find some "healthy" frozen entrees—great "fallback" meal insurance, if you like how they taste (check labels to ensure they're really "healthy," and watch the sodium). Pick up some 100 percent fruit juice concentrates and, for semi-indulgent treats, stock up on low-fat ice milks, yogurts and/or sorbets. Look for single-serving packages that allow you to eat a fixed amount.

Canned/Packaged Food: While these sections can be a minefield of temptations, there are plenty of healthy staples to be found. Choose whole-grain pastas (there are some astonishingly tasty brands now available) and brown rice, as well as "quick" whole grains like whole-wheat couscous, quinoa and quick-cooking barley. Look for canned fruits packed in water or their own juices, and vegetables canned without salt. For convenient protein fixes, try canned beans, water-packed tuna, canned salmon and sardines—and reduced-sodium soups based on broth or beans.

> "When I buy cookies I eat just four and throw the rest away. But first I spray them with Raid so I won't dig them out of the garbage later. Be careful, though, because that Raid really doesn't taste that bad."
>
> JANETTE BARBER, COMEDIAN

Looking for a good salad dressing? Focus on flavor rather than worrying too much about the fat content, since the whole point of dressing is to get you to eat more salads. "Reduced-fat" and "fat-free" dressings often contain similar amounts of calories and might not be worth the flavor trade-off. Don't forget to pick up some interesting vinegars, which add calorie-free flavor to just about anything; try balsamic, sherry and apple cider vinegars.

In the cereal aisle, seek out brands labeled "whole-grain" (with whole grains as the first ingredient) and with at least 8 grams of fiber per serving. Check the label to avoid added sugars; you can always add sweetness with your own sliced fresh fruit. In the snack section, best options include whole-grain snack crackers, whole-wheat pretzels, brown rice cakes, whole-grain crispbreads and popcorn (choose "light" microwave variety or—even better—pop it yourself in an air popper or on the stove, in a heart-healthy oil like peanut or canola).

Bakery: Since sandwich bread is a staple, be choosy: you'll want one that gives you plenty of whole grains in a tasty package. Look for breads, English muffins, bagels and rolls labeled "100 percent whole-wheat," with at least 3 grams of fiber apiece (the first ingredient in the list should begin with the word "whole"). Try "lunch"-size rolls for burgers and sandwiches; you'll get a more reasonable portion. Store bread in the freezer to keep it fresher longer; just thaw on the counter as needed. Whole-wheat versions of pita and flour tortillas can usually be found here, too, along with corn tortillas; keep them to a 7-inch diameter or less.

Among the cookies and cakes, best choices for a splurge are those in bite-size portions, such as brownie bites, mini muffins or flavored meringues. Be wary of "fat-free" bakery treats, which often have as many or even more calories than their "regular" counterparts. Don't waste your calories on anything that doesn't taste fabulous.

note: the DVs are set according to how many calories you eat—and labels usually use 2,000 to 2,500 calories as a reference, which is probably more than your calorie goal for weight loss. If you're only eating 1,500 calories daily, for example, your DV goals will be approximately one-fourth to one-third lower than what's on the label.

Leave a bite behind. Even if it's just a forkful of potato, a little bit left on your plate will remind you that there's still food available, and you don't need to eat it.

TRIGGER FOODS

With this plan there are no forbidden foods. We believe that creating a "Never Eat" stigma just makes the off-limits food even more desirable—and actually increases the chances you'll break down and eat it.

> **It is not the great temptations that ruin us; it is the little ones.**
>
> JOHN W. DEFOREST,
> CIVIL WAR NOVELIST

Nonetheless, there's no denying that everyone has "trigger" foods they have a hard time controlling. For some, it's pizza: they can't stop at just one slice. Others can't enjoy just a scoop of ice cream as long as there's more in the freezer. There are many reasons why foods like these can set us off, and we'll talk more about them in Chapter 4. But for now, it's helpful to know what they are, so you can decide how to deal with them.

Successful weight losers know they must face their triggers head on. Here are some techniques they've used to cope:

Limit trigger foods to an occasional treat. Erin's family goes out for pizza once a month, when she enjoys two slices of her favorite sausage-mushroom pie.

Eat single-serving portions. Jeff loves ice cream, but finds it easier to stay in control if he has small, individually wrapped ice cream sandwiches in his freezer.

Enjoy them "off site." Steve can't imagine Sunday breakfast without glazed chocolate doughnuts. But he no longer buys a boxful at the supermarket, knowing he can't resist their siren song from the kitchen. Instead, he takes himself to the doughnut store and just orders one.

Decide on what you can forgo without missing it. Martha gave up spreading cream cheese on her morning muffin. She found that as long as the muffin was warm out of the oven, she didn't feel deprived.

NOW YOU TRY IT:

Look at your food diary and see if you can identify some of your biggest trigger foods. List them below, then use the space that follows to come up with a strategy for handling each.

My food triggers: **Coping strategies:**

_____   _____

_____   _____

_____   _____

_____   _____

_____   _____

CHECK-IN: YOUR FOOD STRENGTHS AND CHALLENGES

Every day you make dozens of decisions about what, when and how much you're going to eat. Take some time now to evaluate the skills you already have to make those decisions, and those areas that need extra work.

First, focus on your strengths—those skills that can work to your advantage. You might love salad—or perhaps you're a great cook. Now, think about how you can capitalize on those pluses with real actions: Could you aim to have salad for dinner at least three times a week? Or experiment with a new, enlightened recipe each week (like the ones in this book)? List some of your food strengths and strategies here.

MY FOOD STRENGTH #1: _____

I'LL USE THAT STRENGTH TO MY ADVANTAGE BY: _____

MY FOOD STRENGTH #2: _____

I'LL USE THAT STRENGTH TO MY ADVANTAGE BY: _____

MY FOOD STRENGTH #3: _____

I'LL USE THAT STRENGTH TO MY ADVANTAGE BY: _____

Now, think about the food patterns and habits that are getting in the way of your eating the way you want to. Perhaps you don't think a meal is complete without dessert (even breakfast). Or you hate any green vegetable. Again, think of some specific actions you can take to get around these challenges. A green-vegetable hater might try including a nongreen vegetable—say, carrots, tomatoes or cauliflower—at every lunch and dinner, and the dessert lover could try switching to decaffeinated hazelnut coffee for an end-of-meal treat.

MY FOOD CHALLENGE #1: _____

I'LL WORK AROUND THAT CHALLENGE BY: _____

MY FOOD CHALLENGE #2: _____

I'LL WORK AROUND THAT CHALLENGE BY: _____

MY FOOD CHALLENGE #3: _____

I'LL WORK AROUND THAT CHALLENGE BY: _____

CHAPTER 3
MAKE THE RIGHT MOVES

MOVING MORE IS THE SECRET WEAPON FOR WEIGHT LOSS—AND FOR LIFE

So many popular diets try to tiptoe around the topic of exercise, or pay it token lip service, but the fact is that exercise—even light exercise—makes weight loss much easier. Even more important, move more and your lost weight is much more likely to stay lost.

Losing weight, we know, is all about balancing energy—that is, balancing calories. Until now, we've focused on just one side of that simple equation: energy in, or the calories you eat and drink daily. In this chapter, we shift to the other side of the ledger: energy out, or the calories you burn through activity. You know the drill by now: when we burn more calories than we consume, we lose weight. We can create this negative calorie balance either by cutting back on how much we eat or by boosting our daily activity level. Again, the best strategy is to do both.

Studies show that making a regular commitment to being active is the best predictor of long-term success in a weight-loss program. Just look at the 5,000-plus successful "losers" in the National Weight Control Registry, who have lost a minimum of 30 pounds or more and kept it off for at least a year. While they've used countless different methods to lose the pounds, one common thread unites virtually all of them: engaging in regular physical activity.

> "I've gone from being pretty sedentary to walking about four miles every day. That's just been a real gradual buildup. I'm almost surprised to hear myself say I walk four miles a day, because I never thought I'd do that in my life."
>
> —Gail, 53 (50 pounds lost)

> **"**Just 'cause you got the monkey off your back doesn't mean the circus has left town. **"**
>
> GEORGE CARLIN, COMEDIAN

Clearly, keeping active is a critical factor in helping lost weight stay off for good. That's the conclusion of a major follow-up study of HMO members who'd completed a weight-loss program: months after the program ended, researchers compared people who'd managed to keep the pounds off with those who had gained them back. The main difference? Almost all the maintainers (90 percent) still exercised regularly, while only about a third of the weight regainers still did.

So if you truly want to lose weight once and for all, you will need to make a commitment to living a more active life. But the good news is, you can do it—no matter where you're at now.

STEP 5: COMMIT TO MOVE MORE

I don't believe in "magic bullets," but when it comes to making a weight-loss program more effective, regular physical activity comes pretty close. Besides burning calories—which makes it easier to achieve that all-important negative calorie balance that leads to weight loss—exercise also helps curb appetite. It works by slowing the movement of food throughout your digestive system so you feel full longer. Becoming more physically fit

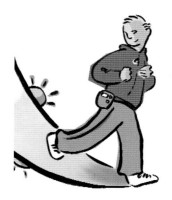

makes your body more effective at burning off calories, even when you're not moving. (And of course, it's not easy to eat ice cream when you're running.)

We used to think that a little weight "creep-up" was an inevitable part of getting older. But now we know it doesn't have to be that way; staying active can help stave off the "inevitable" increase in fat as we age. In a recent study of over 41,500 women runners, those who ran the most tended to gain the least amount of body fat as they aged. And it's definitely not too late to make a difference: exercise's effect on reducing body fat tended to increase with age.

FIRST, THE BASICS

There are two main types of physical activity and both play an important role in managing your weight and keeping you healthy:

Lifestyle exercise—movement that is part of your regular routine, like lifting groceries, doing household chores, moving around at work and of course the walking you do to get to and from those places.

Programmed exercise—activity meant specifically as exercise. Programmed exercise has no other purpose than to make you healthier and fitter, help you manage your weight and (hopefully) be fun. A daily walk or run, workouts at the health club or participation in sports all fit into this category.

Ideally, you will decide to work on boosting your amount of both lifestyle and programmed activity, but our main focus will be on getting you to work regular, programmed exercise into your life. We've found that making this intentional commitment to an exercise routine is the best way to make sure being active is a lifelong habit.

At what pace is moderately intense activity? It should make you breathe harder and have some difficulty talking, but you should still be able to carry on a conversation.

It Just Feels Good

Many people shy away from "exercise" because they think it will leave them tired and out of breath. But as you gradually progress to being more active, just the opposite happens: you'll feel more energized and empowered. Just think what it will do to your self-confidence as you're able to achieve goals that used to exhaust you: climbing stairs without huffing and puffing, or being able to carry a toddler on your back without breaking into a sweat. No wonder older people who exercise regularly say they have a greater sense of well-being and "self-efficacy" than those who don't.

Keeping active might also make you happier. Regular aerobic exercise can help stimulate production of endorphins, "feel-good" chemicals in the brain—that's what's behind the "runner's high" some athletes experience. But you don't have to be an elite athlete to get a boost, either; studies show that regular activity, including walking and strength training, can improve mood and reduce stress. It can also help you get a good night's sleep, sometimes as effectively as taking a sleeping pill. People who exercise regularly tend to fall asleep quicker and stay asleep longer. What's not to love?

CHOOSE YOUR REGIMEN

Any exercise that gets your large muscle groups moving, like walking, running or biking, is excellent for managing your weight. These so-called aerobic exercises get your heart and lungs going, so they're tops in burning calories and building your stamina.

We recommend walking as your main form of programmed exercise. Why? There's no other exercise routine that's quite as simple and accommodating to any lifestyle. In fact, it's already part of your lifestyle. You already know how to do it, and you don't have to buy any special equipment other than a pair of comfortable, supportive walking shoes. You can walk alone or with others, at any time of day, indoors or out. Mile for mile, it burns almost as many calories as running does, with less stress on your joints. How long you go is more important than how far you go.

Other good choices for aerobic exercise are jumping rope, cross-country skiing or using rowing machines or elliptical trainers. You might also choose organized activities, such as an aerobics or dance class. Just be sure you can attend them regularly, and that you're moving continuously throughout your session.

JOIN THE TEAM. (AGAIN.)

Team sports like soccer, baseball and tennis are a terrific way to make a regular commitment to being active. Moreover, they make fitness fun and social, which just might be the incentive you need to get started. You're also more motivated to show up when you know a team, or a partner, is waiting for you.

Don't worry if you haven't been on a team since high school; chances are, there's a recreational league that welcomes participants at all levels. For information, check out your neighborhood recreation center or continuing education program, or the YMCA. Have fun!

TICK, TICK, TICK: THE POWER OF THE PEDOMETER

Need a little push to get you started moving regularly? Consider investing in a pedometer or step counter. This little wearable device tracks the number of steps you take daily—every single step, including walking down the hall to the bathroom and going to the mailbox. It can be powerfully motivating to see how many steps you've taken by the end of the day, and how easy it is to add a few more.

While most of us can easily fit in an additional thousand daily steps without having to become serious walkers, most step-counting advocates suggest aiming much higher. A good starting goal is about 2,000 daily steps—that adds up

---

Exercise Lite

You've probably heard the advice of public health and fitness experts, such as the Centers for Disease Control (CDC) and The American College of Sports Medicine, recommending that all of us try to accumulate at least 30 minutes of physical activity throughout the day, most (if not all) days of the week.

While that may sound like a tall order if you're not active now, keep in mind that just about any activity counts, as long as it gets your heart rate up and your breath coming faster—whether it's vacuuming or raking leaves (see "Calories Burned in 10 Minutes," page 54). And you don't have to do it all at once, either; studies show that for weight loss and fitness gains, accumulating short bursts of activity throughout the day—say, a 10-minute walk in the morning, a five-minute jog up and down stairs during your lunch break and 15 minutes of walking the dog in the evening—is as effective as doing it all in one 30-minute session. Some people might find those small bits easier to work into a busy schedule too.

All that is good advice, and a great way to get you started on the path to becoming more active. But do try to work toward the goal of making a commitment to at least 30 minutes of programmed activity daily. It's the simplest way to make sure you've met your activity goals and, in the long run, a regular routine is much easier to make plans around.

to about one mile. Work up gradually, increasing your steps by about 500 per week, until you've reached what many consider the ideal goal of 10,000 steps daily, the equivalent of five miles.

A good pedometer doesn't have to be expensive; a reliable model will cost about $20 to $30. (Not long ago, a major fast-food chain was even giving them out for free with a "healthy" meal combo!) For the motivation it delivers, it's well worth the investment.

STRENGTH TRAINING

While aerobic activities are most effective for calorie burning, another kind is also important for building fitness: strength training, or resistance training. This type of exercise involves using your muscles to push or pull weight by lifting weights, working out on weight machines or using resistance bands or stability balls. Resistance exercises like pushups and abdominal crunches also qualify, because the weight you're pushing and pulling against is your own.

Strength training helps strengthen bones and muscles and improves your body's sense of balance. It also revs up your metabolism; muscle tissue burns calories, so the more you have, the more calories you'll burn. And, as you're losing weight, strength training helps preserve some muscle tissue that might otherwise be lost along with the fat.

One of the best reasons to add strength training to your exercise routine, though, is that it produces satisfying results fairly quickly. No matter how old or sedentary you are, you'll soon notice that everyday tasks, like lifting groceries, are easier to do. This can give your weight-loss plan a motivating kick start.

You don't have to be a pumped-up bodybuilder or gym rat to benefit from strength training: as little as 15 minutes a day, two or three days a week, is usually enough to produce noticeable fitness gains. It doesn't take a large investment in equipment—just a pair of inexpensive hand weights can be used for a wide range of strength-building exercises. (Instructional guides are available at bookstores and online.) To get started on a strength-training program, you may want to ask your doctor for a recommendation or check your local YMCA, neighborhood recreation center or health club. If you're trying it for the first time, it's worth investing in a few sessions with an exercise trainer;

5 Ways to Become a Walkaholic: Tips from Walking Pros

Always be ready. Keep a pair of walking shoes and socks at work and by the door at home, so an impromptu stroll is easy.

Dress right. Choose loose, comfortable clothing that gives you plenty of room to move your arms and legs. A good pair of walking or running shoes, with socks, is also a must. They don't have to be expensive—but don't skimp on comfort to save a few pennies, either. (Just think of walking shoes as your cheapest form of health insurance.) Replace your shoes when they become worn down.

Enrich the experience. Listen to your favorite music while you work out—research suggests it will help you stick with your regimen longer. Or try talk radio, podcasts or books on CD. You can also make your walks a destination in themselves, by trying a new course every once in a while—perhaps a local park, lake path or arboretum instead of your usual neighborhood walk.

Mall-walk. Indoor walking eliminates the "bad-weather" excuse and it's a great place to meet a friend and socialize as you move. To avoid temptations to buy at the stores (not to mention the fiendishly aromatic cinnamon buns at the food court), leave your wallet and credit cards behind.

Find a walking partner. Besides having someone to talk to and make the walk more interesting, a partner helps make you more accountable. You'll be less likely to skip a walk if you know someone's waiting for you. If you feel unsafe or self-conscious walking alone, a partner can make all the difference. Need help finding a partner? Check your local mall or neighborhood recreation center for walking-club information.

those that are certified as athletic trainers, strength and conditioning coaches or personal trainers are your best bet.

IN CASE YOU NEED MORE CONVINCING...

If losing weight, having more energy and looking and feeling great aren't incentive enough to get you moving more, just think about how happy it will make your doctor. There are literally dozens of medical reasons why exercise is probably one of the most important things you can do for your health. Studies show that regular physical activity can:

• Keep your heart healthy by strengthening your heart muscle and making it more efficient, lowering blood pressure and boosting your levels of heart-friendly HDLs (high-density lipoproteins).

• Help reduce risks of some types of chronic diseases, including breast cancer and some aggressive forms of prostate cancer. If you have diabetes or are "borderline," regular exercise can improve your blood-sugar control. Got arthritis? Strength training and aerobic exercise might help boost flexibility and strength.

• Keep your brain sharp. Regular exercise helps improve blood flow to the brain, and regular exercisers tend to do better in maintaining cognitive ability as they age.

• Help you live longer. A recent report from the long-term Framingham Heart Study—which has been gathering health data from more than 5,000 people for almost six decades—found that those participants who had moderate or high levels of activity lived 1.3 or 3.7 years longer, respectively, than those who were mostly sedentary.

TRACK YOURSELF TO SEE YOURSELF

However you choose to become more active, you'll need to make changes in your daily habits. And one of the most powerful tools for mastering those changes is something you're already doing with your eating plan: keeping a diary. In the same way that a food diary helps make you aware of (and accountable for) what you eat, an activity diary can help you build more activity into your days.

Self-tracking is self-motivating, especially if you think of yourself as a "nonexerciser." By writing down each time you get moving, you give yourself credit for being active— and each activity adds up!

You can start right now with the Activity Log on page 238, which you can photocopy to keep on hand. In it,

---

Doing It Right: 2 Essential Guidelines for Any Kind of Exercise

◆ **Take it easy.** Don't overdo your workout sessions; you're bound to end up feeling stiff and sore tomorrow, and there's nothing more demotivating. Instead, proceed at a rate that feels comfortable but challenging, and slow down or stop if you're feeling exhausted.

◆ **Warm up and cool down.** Always begin your exercise session with a five-minute warmup to prepare your muscles, lungs and heart for the transition to higher speed or more effort. Likewise, take the last five minutes of your workout for a cooldown to unwind. The easiest way to warm up or cool down is to do your planned activity at a slower pace. Say, if you're walking briskly or running, start and end with five minutes of slower walking. Or hit a few balls against the wall or lightly jog in place before starting your tennis game. Before starting strength training, warm up by doing a series of stretching and bending exercises.

you'll find space to list all your daily activities, the time and duration of each, as well as space to write any thoughts or feelings. Were you feeling great? Exhausted? Did you enjoy it? Knowing your feelings and energy levels can help you plan future activities; if you felt especially energized after a 7 a.m. walk, for example, but exhausted from an after-work stroll, you can schedule future walks for the morning slot.

Starting today, take a few minutes to write down—and give yourself credit for—any heart-pumping activity you've completed. It's most rewarding to do it right after you finish, while it's still fresh in your mind. Here's what a typical day might look like.

Today's Date _____

TIME	ACTIVITY	DURATION/LENGTH	NOTES	CALORIES BURNED
7:15	Walked to office	20 min. / 1 mi.	Tired at first, then energized	
12:30	Walked to drugstore & back	5 min. / ¼ mi.		
6:45	After-dinner bike ride	20 min. / 4 mi.	Felt great, but got hungry passing the ice cream store— change route next time	

TOTAL EXERCISE MINUTES: _____   TOTAL CALORIES BURNED: _____

WHAT ABOUT CALORIES?

There's also a space on your Activity Log to estimate the calories you burned off with your activity. You don't have to worry about this the first week of keeping your log—just concentrate on writing everything down and learning from what you've noted about yourself.

But next week, start making an effort to track your exercise calories too. It's terrifically motivating to add up all the calories you're losing—and to see your progress in becoming fitter.

How many calories can you burn off as you move? It depends on your size. People of different weights burn calories at different rates (after all, it takes more work to move a 200-pound weight than a 150-pound one). Use the "Calories Burned in 10 Minutes" chart, page 54, to help you calculate. Or, to keep things simple, you can also apply the following inexact but good general rules of thumb:

• Walking or running one mile is equal to 100 calories burned.
• Riding a bike for the same amount of time it takes you to walk one mile burns about 100 calories. (Biking burns fewer calories than walking, since the bike carries your weight, not you. So you'll need to bicycle farther to burn the same number of calories.)

CALORIES BURNED IN 10 MINUTES

1. Find your weight (use the lower weight category that most closely matches your weight).
2. Estimate your activity into 10-minute units.
3. Multiply units by calories expended (for your weight) in 10 minutes of exercise. For example, if you weigh 160 pounds and jog/walked for 20 minutes: multiply 2 (units) x 68 calories (calories expended in 10 minutes for a 150-pound person). Your approximate caloric expenditure is 136 calories for your 20-minute activity.

ACTIVITY	125 pounds	150 pounds	175 pounds	200 pounds	225 pounds
Bicycling, leisurely 10 mph	38	45	53	61	68
Bicycling, 10-12 mph (light)	57	68	80	91	102
Bicycling, mountain (strenuous)	80	97	113	129	145
Bicycling, stationary	66	80	93	106	119
Canoeing/rowing for pleasure	33	40	46	53	60
Football or baseball, playing catch	24	28	33	38	43
Gardening	47	57	66	76	85
Golf, pulling clubs	47	57	73	76	85
Golf, power cart	33	40	46	53	60
Health Club stair machine/treadmill	85	102	119	136	153
Household chores, light	24	28	33	38	43
Household chores, moderate	38	45	53	61	68
Jog/walk combination	57	68	80	91	102
Jogging, general	66	80	93	106	119
Running, 5 mph, 12-minute mile	76	91	106	121	136
Skating, ice, 9 mph	52	62	73	83	94
Skiing, downhill, moderate effort	57	68	80	91	102
Skiing, x-country, light/moderate	76	91	106	121	136
Soccer, casual	66	80	93	106	119
Stretching or yoga	24	28	33	38	43
Swimming leisurely (not laps)	57	68	80	91	102
Swimming laps, freestyle	66	80	93	106	119
Tennis, doubles	66	68	80	91	102
Walking, 3 mph, moderate pace	31	37	44	50	56
Walking, very brisk pace	47	57	66	76	85
Water aerobics	38	45	53	61	68
Weight lifting, moderate	28	34	40	45	51

Values calculated from University of Vermont Dept. of Nutrition & Food Sciences, and from Nieman, D.C.: Exercise Testing and Prescription 6th edition, © 2006, McGraw Hill.

NOW YOU TRY IT: ADDING IT ALL UP

Complete the calories column in the sample Activity Log (page 53) for a 150-pound person (who walks at a moderate pace and bikes 12 mph), and total them up—along with the exercise minutes total—at the end of the day.

Answers to "NOW YOU TRY IT"

Total Calories Burned: 229

Total Exercise Minutes: 45

How much programmed activity should you aim for? A good goal is to target burning 1,000 calories per week in programmed exercise. If you can walk a mile in 20 minutes, 1,000 calories in programmed activity is the weekly equivalent of walking 10 miles. (So, if you walk for 30 minutes each day, you will be right about where you want to be with about 1,050 calories burned.)

If you're not regularly active now, phase yourself into the habit gradually by setting this week's goal at 250 calories or 2.5 miles. Every 2 weeks, raise your goal by 250 calories, until you've reached the goal of 1,000 calories per week.

> If you didn't get any extra activity on a given day, don't forget to write it down in your activity log, too, and the feelings that may have led to your decision to sit out that day. Later on, you might be able to spot patterns that can help you confront—and overcome—those feelings, next time they come to call.

REALITY CHECK: MORE IS BETTER

While 1,000 calories a week in programmed exercise will help you achieve your weight-loss goals, you might want to think of this as a starting point: recent research suggests that more exercise may be necessary to maintain a weight loss and prevent weight gain. In fact, those "successful losers" we mentioned in the National Weight Control Registry report burned about 2,800 calories in exercise, on average, each week. And, when researchers compare results when people are given exercise goals of burning 1,000 calories or 2,500 calories, they've found that those in the higher-goal groups tend to maintain their weight loss longer. When it comes to exercise, then, more is definitely better.

But don't lose heart and quit before you start. Remember, any exercise is good, and any activity is always better than the sedentary lifestyle most Americans lead. Moreover, once you're on the path to being more active, you'll likely be able to move on to higher exercise goals with ease. After all, most of those successful "losers" had to start somewhere too.

CAN I EAT MORE IF I EXERCISE MORE?

While it's motivating to know about how many calories exercise can burn, it's not a good idea to think of exercise calories and food calories as trade-off items. Doing this can lead to some pretty silly bargaining: for example, "If I run three miles, I can eat another doughnut." Most of us underestimate how many calories we eat anyway—and that includes us dietitians, even though we try our best. I tell our weight-loss program participants not to think of physical activity as a way of burning off food, but as a way to compensate for those extra calories they might have overlooked or underestimated throughout the day.

NOW YOU TRY IT: YOUR FAVORITE MOVES

Write down the different types of programmed exercise you've tried over the years. Write down next to each one how you felt about that activity. Did you enjoy it? Hate it? Why? Knowing these feelings can help point you to patterns in your thinking about exercise, and help you decide which activities are going to work best for you.

Activities I've Tried /Liked/Disliked   **Why?**

_____   _____

_____   _____

_____   _____

_____   _____

_____   _____

_____   _____

Now, think about the activities you've never tried but always had an interest in doing.

Activities I haven't tried but would like to:

_____

_____

_____

_____

_____

_____

_____

_____

_____

_____

_____

Now, set your goals.

Try at least one new activity each week—or add an activity you've enjoyed in the past but haven't done for a while. Write them on the first page of your Activity Log, so you'll always have them in sight. This will help you find a variety of activities you enjoy and can use as part of your programmed exercise routine.

Activity I'll Try This Week: _____

_____

_____

LIFESTYLE EXERCISE

Up until now, we've focused on intentional, programmed exercise to schedule into your day. But there is plenty to be gained, and pounds to be lost, by making small changes in your daily routine. If you're like most Americans, your daily routine is, well, pretty sedentary. In our modern society, it's hard not to be. Between driving to work, taking elevators and escalators to move around the building, sitting at computers all day, and coming home to TV and the Internet at night, there aren't many opportunities to move your body. It's up to you to invent a few reasons.

Think about what your day is like and how you can burn a few extra calories here and there. Can you use the upstairs bathroom when you're downstairs, for example? Do toe raises while you're washing dishes? Each one of these extra activities doesn't make a big dent in your daily routine, but keeps you in the "calorie-burning" mindset. Every time you repeat them, you're doing something positive for yourself—and that can be hugely empowering.

Don't forget to record these "lifestyle" activities in your activity log. Though they don't count toward your weekly exercise goal, every move you make is helpful. And, having a bank of extra activity "credits" helps compensate for when you've overestimated how many calories you've burned through programmed exercise. Just as we tend to underestimate how much we eat, we're usually a little too optimistic when we estimate our physical-activity levels: most people overestimate by about 50 percent!

> **" It's easier to go down a hill than up it but the view is much better at the top. "**
>
> HENRY WARD BEECHER, MINISTER AND EDUCATOR

---

6 Ways to Sneak Lifestyle Exercise Into Your Day

Think of this as stealth exercise: doing what you're doing now, only being more active at it.

• Follow the "five and 10" rule for escalators and elevators: Take the stairs if you only need to go up five floors or less, or down 10 floors or less. Walk on the escalator rather than just standing there.

• Walk to errands less than a mile away whenever possible. When you do take motorized transportation, park in the farthest-away spot in the parking lot, or get off one stop earlier on the train or bus.

• Change classes. Remember the four minutes' time between classes in high school, to switch rooms? Reinstate them. Every hour or so, take four minutes to move around: get some water, use the restroom, walk to someone's office with a message or question, rather than calling or e-mailing them. Set an alarm on your watch or computer screen if you need a reminder.

• Don't be so darn efficient. Make several trips up and down stairs to bring up laundry, take out garbage, tote cleaning supplies, etc. Do one errand at a time, making a separate trip (preferably on foot or bike) for each one.

• Keep moving. When watching TV, do situps, leg lifts or lift light weights during commercials. When watching your kids at sports games or practice, use that time to walk or jog around the field.

• Fire the lawn guy. Mowing your own lawn and doing your own weeding all burn calories. The same goes for vacuuming, window washing and other housekeeping chores. (Why not use the money you saved to get a new pair of walking shoes or a snazzy track outfit?)

WHAT'S STOPPING YOU?

Everyone has them: reasons why you can't—or won't—get into a regular exercise routine. Here are a few of my favorites, and some ways you can face them head on:

"I don't have enough time."
• Break exercise into smaller segments rather than taking it all in one chunk (see "Exercise Lite," page 50).
• Multitask—do crunches while watching TV, or jog in place while you're on hold on the telephone.
• Adjust your schedule. Get up a half-hour earlier so you can get a walk in before the kids wake up, for example.
• Make it a nonnegotiable routine. Mark off a chunk of time during your day that's inviolate—say, the lunch hour at work—and let everyone know you're not available during that time. Yes, things will come up, but you'll fit in a workout more often than not.

"I'm too embarrassed/afraid to exercise."
• Bring a friend along on your walks for moral support. Try a new neighborhood where you're not likely to run into anyone you know.
• Work out at home with an exercise or dance DVD.
• Try a gym that feels comfortable and friendly—many aren't the hard-body havens you may be imagining. Most welcome all sizes, ages and fitness levels.

"Exercise is too hard."
• Take it slow and steady. Start with a comfortable amount of activity and work up gradually, adding a few more minutes each day. This isn't a race, this is life!
• If it feels bad, stop. Listen to your body; exercise shouldn't cause you pain. Don't exercise to the point of exhaustion; you should always be able to carry on a conversation throughout.
• Keep going. If you've got minor muscle aches from overexertion, take it easier the next day, but don't stop altogether. Getting some kind of gentle movement actually helps your muscles recover better from stiffness and soreness than going "cold turkey."

> "I used to run into people who would say, 'I can't stand not getting exercise for a couple of days,' and I'd say, 'Yeah, right. Why on earth would you really enjoy it?' But it really does get into your system... after three weeks following the program, exercise felt good and I actually started craving it."
> —**John**, 50 (75 pounds lost)

"Exercise doesn't work for me."
• Correction: You just haven't found the right kind of exercise yet. Focus on adding more lifestyle exercise to your day, and be sure to count it in your activity log. Every effort you make to move more counts.

Remember, what's past is past. You may have had some bad experiences with fitness in the past (say, an overbearing gym teacher), but you're on a different path now. Pay attention to the feelings and thoughts you write in your food diary and activity log—they can help you see a way around your exercise demons.

> ❝ My grandmother started walking five miles a day when she was sixty. She's ninety-three today and we don't know where the hell she is. ❞
>
> ELLEN DEGENERES, COMEDIAN

CHECK-IN: LIVING MORE ACTIVELY

- **Stephen paces the room while talking on the phone.**

- **Carolyn walks the neighbor's dog.**

- **Edward "unplugged" his kitchen so that he uses elbow grease instead of an electrically powered gadget to beat eggs, chop vegetables, shred cheese and other cooking tasks.**

How can you incorporate more lifestyle activity into your days? Make a list of at least four ways, and be creative! Aim to include at least two of these activities each day.

I CAN ADD MORE ACTIVITY INTO MY DAY BY:

1 _____

2 _____

3 _____

4 _____

5 _____

6 _____

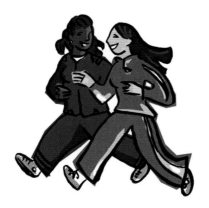

CHAPTER 4

TAKE ON THE TRIP-UPS

TO BECOME A SUCCESSFUL WEIGHT LOSER, YOU MUST FIRST BECOME A PLANNER. EXPECT—AND PREPARE FOR—LAPSES BY GETTING THE SUPPORT YOU NEED.

Some days, it can seem like a conspiracy. Something arises to thwart your best intentions to eat right and move more. On really bad days, it may seem that everything is working against you. Here are a few typical day-after explanations and regrets from participants in our weight-loss programs:

- "There were only fast-food restaurants at the airport, so I had to have a burger and fries for dinner."

- "I couldn't go running today because we had a day-long training session at work."

- "I wasn't really hungry, but when that pizza commercial came on, I just had to go out and get a slice. Actually, it was three slices."

- "I was going to have salad for dinner, but my best friend called and wanted to go out for Chinese food."

- "Aunt Judy served us her famous noodle kugel. How could I say no to that?"

The best way to handle disruptions like these is to expect them—they do happen to everyone—and be ready to handle them. By taking the next key step—getting support—you can put workable plans in place so that a temporary lapse doesn't turn into a long-term slide.

We'll start by looking at those situations that trigger you to eat more, and arm you to fight back with classic techniques of behavior modification. Then, we'll tackle those challenges life throws your way—restaurants, holiday parties, traveling and more—with strategies for handling them with ease. Along the way, we'll show you how to get the support you need, from others and, most importantly, from yourself.

> "Success is to be measured not so much by the position that one has reached in life as by the obstacles which he has overcome."
>
> BOOKER T. WASHINGTON, POLITICAL LEADER & EDUCATOR

NAME YOUR TRIGGERS

What makes you eat? Each of us has different eating triggers, and some might be more obvious than others. (Rereading your food journal is one excellent way to spot occasions and foods that tend to trip you up.) Learning to recognize your own eating cues will help you figure out how to manage them better, so let's take a look:

Certain places or actions. Walking in the door when you get home from work, sitting down in front of the TV or even sitting in a particular comfortable chair can be powerful "feed me!" triggers. Or perhaps you can't talk on the phone or read the newspaper without having something to nibble. However it began, you may have come to associate those activities with eating a snack.

Seeing and/or smelling food. Tantalizing aromas and seductive visuals of food can get your digestive juices flowing and activate your "hunger" meter. Some people seem to be more susceptible to these cues than others. If walking by a pizzeria or a doughnut shop gets your senses reeling, you might be one of these food "hyper-responders."

Boredom. If you've got downtime or are busy with a task that doesn't command your full attention, you might crave food simply to have something engaging to do. Going to get something to eat might feel like switching channels to a better station.

Emotions. While some people react to stressful or unpleasant situations by losing appetite, many people find themselves eating more to help them cope. It's easy to see why: food is pleasurable and comforting, and after all, eating is one major way we care for ourselves. Overeating can even produce a drowsy calm (some call it a "food coma") that can be quite soothing. The act of eating itself can be a distraction, too, if you're a procrastinator: ever wonder why you're longing to cook up a delicious, complicated dinner when you have a deadline looming?

Research shows that positive emotions can trigger overeating, too. You might find yourself eating more when you're celebrating an accomplishment, anticipating a happy event or falling in love, for example.

> **❝** If it weren't for Philo T. Farnsworth, inventor of television, we'd still be eating frozen radio dinners. **❞**
>
> JOHNNY CARSON,
> COMEDIAN

BEHAVIOR MODIFICATION 101

No matter what gets you hungry, behavior modification can be a powerful tool in turning things around. Here are a few basic concepts, and how you can put them to work.

Conditioning. When you practice two or more behaviors simultaneously—like watching TV and snacking—you can eventually associate one with the other, even if the two have nothing to do with each other. (Think of the experiments behavioral research pioneer Ivan Pavlov conducted in the early 1900s: he conditioned dogs to expect food every time they heard a bell ring, simply by regularly ringing a bell just before feeding time.) In effect, you have conditioned yourself to expect a reward (food) with a particular action (TV watching). So in order to break

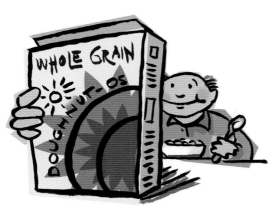

the behavior, you need to break the chain of events that lead from one situation to the other—disassociating eating from the activity. How to separate eating from TV? You could change the setting, by moving the television to another room. Or switch to another, less comfortable chair that makes eating awkward. You could simply outlaw food from the TV room. Again, it is a fundamental good rule to eat only in one designated place in the house. Ideally, it is sitting down at the kitchen or dining room table. Pick one place in your house where you will eat and be sure to eat there and only there. (Of course, it has to be a room without the TV.) Likewise, if you've come to associate being stressed-out with heading for the kitchen, try a calming activity that's separate from eating, such as taking a five-minute walk, practicing some deep-breathing exercises or calling a supportive friend.

Stimulus control. This key behavioral concept focuses on making the environment as conducive as possible to the behavior you're seeking; in other words, making it easier to do the right thing. For weight loss, that means trying to control the stimuli or triggers in your environment that make it difficult to follow your eating and exercise plan. Setting up a well-thought-out personal environment to work for you eliminates the need to rely on willpower. (We all know how well willpower works!) When you put your sneakers by your front door so you won't forget to take a daily walk, or store the ready-to-eat carrots front and center in the refrigerator so they're the first thing you see when you're hunting for a snack, you're making stimulus control work for you. Conversely, practicing stimulus control also means minimizing the features in your environment that trigger, or enable, the behavior you're trying to eliminate. You want to make it harder to do the wrong thing. Here's how you might use stimulus control for your trigger situations:

> **❝You can't turn back the clock. But you can wind it up again.❞**
>
> BONNIE PRUDDEN,
> PHYSICAL ACTIVITY ENTHUSIAST
> AND MYOTHERAPIST

> **❝As the Sandwich Islander believes that the strength and valor of the enemy he kills passes into himself, so we gain the strength of the temptations we resist.❞**
>
> RALPH WALDO EMERSON, POET,
> ESSAYIST, PHILOSOPHER

- Cross the street to avoid walking by an aromatic bakery or pizza parlor (one dieter we know discreetly holds her nose). Or choose a different route.

- When the appetizing commercials come on the television, leave the room (say, for a few minutes of stair-walking).

- Store the cookies in the back of the cupboard and the ice cream in the back reaches of the freezer, so you're less likely to see them when you open the door. (Of course, many people find that not having them there at all is the fail-safe method of avoiding known trigger foods.)

- When tempting treats come in eye-catching packaging, transfer them to nondescript storage containers.

Compensation. Instead of trying to change a behavior that's contributing to your weight problem, you can change something else in your planning to make room for it. Let's say you don't want to give up having a regular popcorn fix at your family's weekly "movie night." You could compensate by eating fewer servings of starchy foods that day, or eat more lightly in general, so you have room for a small bag (hold the butter). If you really planned ahead, you might have "banked" some extra calories earlier in the week. Or bring your own bowl so you can measure out and enjoy your own portion.

"I've been putting up with a lot of boring meetings today, so I deserve that ice cream sundae."

When you find yourself falling into the "reward yourself with food" trap, remember this counter thought: "Do I also deserve the hours of extra exercise I'm going to have to do to burn off all those calories?"

NOW, YOU TRY IT: TAME YOUR TRIGGERS

Name three triggers that start your eating engine. For each one, list at least two ways you can help stop them from derailing your weight-loss efforts.

Eating Trigger #1: _____

Prevention Strategies: _____

_____

_____

Eating Trigger #2: _____

Prevention Strategies: _____

_____

_____

Eating Trigger #3: _____

Prevention Strategies: _____

_____

_____

TAKE ON THE CHALLENGES

Everybody who tries to lose weight faces daily challenges that test their resolve. But standing up to problems successfully isn't just a matter of willpower or strength of character. It means understanding that challenges are the norm, not the occasional curve ball. Have your strategies ready and waiting. In this section, you'll work on designing your own tactics for getting through some of the most common daily challenges.

CHALLENGE #1: PERNICIOUS PLATEAUS

You're losing weight at a nice, steady pace, and things are going well...then all of a sudden, the scale doesn't budge. For a week, maybe two or longer, you don't see your weight change, even though you know you're following your eating and exercise program. Are you stuck at that weight forever? Time to panic? Not at all. You've probably just reached a plateau, part of nearly everyone's weight-loss odyssey.

> **❝** Get up every day and try a little harder than the day before. **❞**
>
> EMERIL LAGASSE, CHEF

Generally, in the first few weeks of any reduced-calorie eating plan, you're able to shed pounds more easily because you're getting rid of excess water as your body breaks down fat. But once that extra water is gone, the weight loss can slow down, because you don't have as much fat to lose. Consider it a sign of success: you've completed Phase I of your weight loss. Hold steady for a week or two, and you'll probably be right back in the losing corner.

But if you haven't lost more than a half pound in two weeks or so, it's time to reevaluate your plan. First, make an honest assessment of whether you truly are following your plan. Are you continuing to:

- Write down everything you eat in your food diary?

- Add up the calories daily?

- Get some sort of programmed exercise most days of the week?

- Write down your exercise in your activity log?

- Check your portion sizes, using measuring tools if necessary?

If you answered "no" or just "sometimes" to any of these questions, your plan might need a tune-up. Try these strategies for recharging yourself:

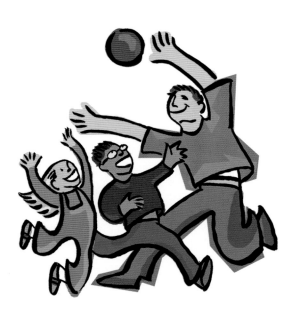

Review your food diary and activity log. Are you consistently forgetting to list some items? Do your comments in the "Notes" section reveal something else at work—say, feeling depressed or stressed? If so, addressing those feelings might help take you out of the plateau.

Get out of your rut. Try a different exercise routine—maybe a dance class or a swim in a local pool. Add intervals to your workout (alternating regular pace with a faster pace). Invite a friend to come along on your next walk, for fresh perspective. Try a new fruit or vegetable next time you're at the supermarket–or experiment with some new recipes (this book is a great start).

Talk with someone who has been there. Know a successful weight loser? Chances are he or she reached a plateau, too, and overcame it. Compare notes, and you just might find a tactic that works for you, along with a healthy dose of inspiration.

Lower your calorie goal slightly—by 75 to 100 calories or so a day, as long as it doesn't bring you below the safe minimum of 1,200 daily calories. Try eating one less serving of a starchy carbohydrate food like white rice or potatoes, or cut out an "extra" like half-and-half in your coffee (or that pat of butter on your muffin).

Bump up your activity a little. For many, this is easier than cutting calories—and it might boost your energy and mood too. Try some "lifestyle exercises" suggested in Chapter 3 (*page 57*), or add five to 10 minutes to your programmed exercise routine. Or, if you aren't doing it already, add strength-training sessions to your fitness routine a couple of times a week.

Get more out of your food diary. Use the "Notes" section to write what's going on and how you're feeling when you eat. Do you find yourself craving potato chips when you've got a big report due? Spooning ice cream from the container when a "good" friend snubs you? Track what you've written, and you might see a pattern. Eventually, you'll be able to link what's going on in your mind with what's going on in your belly.

One proven plateau-buster: For one week, eat only foods for which you know the calorie content. Do not eat any restaurant or take-out food, whose calorie counts are unpredictable. Use your measuring cups and spoons so you know exactly what you're getting, and write down the numbers faithfully in your food diary. It's a bit obsessive (that's why we only recommend one week) but it works!

CHALLENGE #2: HOLIDAYS AND PARTIES

Nobody wants to be a party pooper, but celebrations, holiday and otherwise, can be a major obstacle for anyone watching their weight. Most party fare is, by definition, diet-busting stuff, especially around the holidays. And many holiday traditions center around foods that used to be only once-a-year luxuries for most people, like buttery, sugary cookies. Today, we can have those foods anytime, but we still crave them at holiday gatherings. Trying to eat them moderately can seem positively churlish.

So you're invited to a party? Step one: When you RSVP, ask (politely) what's on the menu. If it sounds like a night of ultra-rich fare, offer to bring a dish to share—something that works with your eating plans, but that you know others will enjoy too. (For ideas, turn to the recipes in the back of this book.) If it's a sit-down affair, ask if you can help serve, so you can have some control over your portion.

Get a (Nonfood) Life

For many of us, food and drink are the context around our social get-togethers. Some social rituals are indelibly intertwined with food: imagine a family reunion without a potluck or a birthday without a cake. Many of us use restaurants and bars as our places to connect with friends, so if you opt out of the eating and drinking, you'll miss out on the bonding. Even if the social occasion isn't about eating, food is almost always offered—or it hovers temptingly in the background, like the concession stand at the movie or ballgame or the snack bar at the golf course.

Socializing without food, then, requires some thinking outside the box. Instead of reserving a table at a restaurant, try scheduling your next get-together with your friends at a place you can walk around, like a museum or an outdoor event like a fair. Consider activities that allow you to chat while you move, like a bike ride, a lake or beachside stroll, or a shopping excursion in a very spread-out mall. And if the gang insists on ordering something to eat, sip a coffee drink instead (nonfat cappuccino is a great way to add a daily milk serving, and it feels like a splurge).

With family get-togethers, try adding some nonfood-oriented elements to the mix. Try a post-meal family walk (rather than family flop-out-in-front-of-the-TV), play charades or start a family story-sharing or scrapbooking session. Yes, it might be awkward at first, but family traditions have to start somehow. And eventually someone— perhaps even your eye-rolling teenage nephew—will thank you for it.

When you get to the party, check out the food offerings and decide on one or two "must-haves"—perhaps the host's specialty dish or a seasonal treat you can't imagine the holidays without. Take a modest portion of each and fill the rest of your plate with vegetables, if you can (there's got to be a veggie platter somewhere). Don't waste calories on calorie-heavy but unremarkable foods you could find anywhere, like potato chips or a standard-issue cheese platter.

Go easy on alcoholic drinks. Alcohol lowers your inhibitions, which can chip away at your resolve to eat mindfully, so that 5-ounce glass of wine might be contributing more than just its own 100 calories. (You must also count those four cheese-stuffed mushroom caps that, after a few sips, became entirely irresistible.) Limit yourself to just one alcoholic drink and nurse it well; the rest of the evening, sip sparkling water with plenty of citrus wedges (add a few drops of grenadine for festive red color if you like).

> "I get a little funny when I'm out of town and I can't have my regular breakfast. I've eaten the same thing for breakfast for a couple of years now:[a whole Montreal-style bagel with a tablespoon of cream cheese]. It's just easier that way. I know it's 240 calories, and it stays with me and it tastes good."
> —**Susannah**, 49 (10 pounds lost)

Above all, focus on the fun, not the food. Enjoy the conversation and the entertainment—and if there's a dance floor, kick up your heels! Laughter, sparkling conversation and mingling all burn calories too.

When you're entertaining, serve up lower-calorie dishes you love, like the recipes in these pages. Consider it an opportunity to open a few people's eyes to what they're missing. No need to announce that it's "lighter" fare, unless someone asks.

CHALLENGE #3: TRAVEL TROUBLE

One of the pleasures (and perils) of travel is depending on your meals being prepared by someone else, and a pretty unavoidable change in your exercise routine. As always, it helps to plan ahead (and never be without a good pair of walking shoes). Try these strategies for staying on track:

Incorporate activity into your trip. Maybe your idea of a great vacation is lying on a beach for a week, but even that plan can accommodate a little movement, as long as it's fun. The next time you plan a vacation or business trip, think about how you can work in some pleasurable activity. Book a walking or bike tour to introduce you to your destination—or use your vacation to try a new sport you've always wondered about, like sea kayaking. Walk the beach each morning and/or evening or amble downtown from your hotel, rather than taking a taxi. Choose entertainment options that keep you moving, like playing mini golf or bowling rather than watching a movie. **Choose the hotel.** Seek out hotels that have health clubs or safe walking routes

5 Airport/Train/Bus Station Fallbacks

• Small slice of plain or vegetable-topped pizza (about 250 calories)*
• Half-sandwich: a pencil-thick layer of turkey breast, lean roast beef or ham, with plenty of lettuce and tomato on whole-wheat, hold the mayo (160 calories)*
• 1 small soft pretzel (210 calories)*
• Kid-size hamburger, hold the fries (284 calories)*
• Small low-fat frozen yogurt with a sprinkle of nuts (156 calories)*

*Calories are estimates.

nearby; call ahead to make sure the "fitness room" isn't just a few ancient exercise bikes. (Pack a jump rope just in case.) If your budget allows, ask for a room with a mini fridge and/or microwave, so you can have some of your meals en suite instead of depending on restaurants or room service. The front-desk staff can point you to the nearest grocery store.

If you're driving, pack a picnic lunch or dinner to eat at a rest stop (save the roadside restaurants for coffee and bathroom stops). For longer trips, take a cooler and stock it with meal-ready nutritious staples—carrots and celery sticks, fresh fruit, bottled water, string cheese, whole-grain crackers. Go over the route ahead of time and plan stopping points for meals: surf the Internet to locate chain restaurants that have healthy menu options. Further browsing can locate alternative road-food sources, like farmers' markets and grocery stores.

On planes, trains and buses, tuck emergency rations in your carry-on bag, if regulations permit, in case of layovers or delays. Use layover/delay time to your advantage: walk around the airport, train or bus station (check your carry-on bag in a locker, if you need to); you might just find an out-of-the-way eatery with healthier offerings that won't blow your calorie budget. But even in the most Spartan of venues you can probably scare up something decent to eat.

> ## 8 Snacks to Pack
>
> - Single-serve applesauce or water-packed canned fruit
> - Fresh fruit
> - String cheese
> - Small bags of high-fiber ready-to-eat cereal
> - Whole-grain crackers
> - Cut-up vegetables (try baby carrots, celery, bell peppers)
> - Energy bars*
> - Small (1-ounce) packages of nuts
>
> ---
>
> * Look for brands providing 225 calories or less, with at least 5 grams of protein, 3 grams of fiber and less than 3 grams of saturated fat per bar.

CHALLENGE #4: NAVIGATING RESTAURANTS

Not so long ago, going to a restaurant for a meal was a big occasion. Today, it's the norm, with Americans spending about half their food dollars in restaurants. Whether you're doing takeout, a fast-food fix or a fancy night out, a well-thought-out plan will save you lots of anxiety, decision-pondering and calories. Here are some calorie-saving strategies that others have found effective:

You choose the restaurant. Select a place whose menu offers healthy options; many now do. If you're not sure, don't hesitate to call ahead and ask. Some restaurants post sample menus online; preview if you can, so you'll know what to expect, and maybe even plan what you'll order. (Have a backup in mind, too, since menus often change more frequently than websites get updated.)

Have a default order. Develop a mental list of fallback meals you can count on no matter what the venue. Just about any restaurant kitchen can serve up at least one of the following lean options: baked chicken or broiled fish with vegetables and a baked potato; pasta with marinara sauce; grilled chicken salad with a healthy vinaigrette dressing (ordered on the side, so you can control the portion).

Decide what's most important. To keep calories down, stick to just one "extra" item in your meal. Enjoy an appetizer or a dessert or a glass of wine—not all three. (Just think of the money you'll save.)

Plan your calories accordingly. Eat lightly at lunch before an evening meal out, or eat smaller, low-calorie meals throughout the day, or even through the week, so that you've banked some extra calories to enjoy at the restaurant. Or, if it's a lunch outing, borrow a few calories from dinner and eat less in the evening.

NOW, YOU TRY IT: ADD SOME MOVES

List 3 ways you could incorporate exercise while you're away from home or traveling.

1. _____
2. _____
3. _____

Don't arrive famished. Otherwise, you'll be tempted to overeat when you're presented with a menu whose main goal is to tantalize—and that's before the bread basket arrives. Instead, have a light snack to take the edge off your hunger—something with a little protein for staying power is ideal. Nibble on a half a protein bar, a few almonds or a piece of string cheese just before you leave for the restaurant.

LIFE IN THE FAST (FOOD) LANE

Opting for a fast-food meal isn't the diet disaster it used to be. For one, fast-food restaurants are now required to post their nutrition information, so you'll know what you're getting. (If you don't see it, ask—or check it out at the restaurant's website first.) And, because they're tuned in to what consumers want, most places now offer some "healthy" options. Take note of these usually smart selections:

- Grilled or roasted chicken sandwiches. Just be sure to ask for no mayonnaise nor (almost-always mayonnaise-based) "special sauce."

- Baked potatoes. Opt for vegetable toppings rather than the cheese and sour cream.

- Deli sandwiches. Skip the cheese and go easy on (or avoid) the mayonnaise; choose roasted lean meats or chicken rather than mayonnaise-rich chicken or tuna salad. Eat the sandwich open-faced, discarding the top bread half if the sandwich is especially large.

- Vegetarian options. Choose vegetable toppings for your pizza, or try a bean burrito or veggie burger.

- Salads. Round out any meal with a "side" or "garden" salad. Some full-meal salads are good options, but croutons and other nonvegetable toppings can quickly pile on the calories. As always, get your dressing on the side.

- Vegetable soup or chili. These are usually filling and relatively low in fat and calories—but not always; check the nutrition information first.

- The kid-size plain burger. This meat portion still satisfies, and it might even come with fruit or carrots.

"My husband and I eat out all the time. I was able to lose weight and go out to dinner all the time—and I drink wine. Twenty years from now I'm going to be drinking a glass of wine at night. I just know that about me, and I'm not going to pretend that I'm not going to do it. So I factored into my planning that I was going to be drinking a glass of wine at night, and that I'd go out to eat. For me, it's making better choices. You don't eat all the bread on the table, or you don't eat the bread. You get some things with vegetables. It's just my lifestyle."

—**Julie**, 47 (45 pounds lost)

STEP 6: GET SUPPORT

Because losing weight can be so challenging, we can't expect to do it alone. In fact, in all my years of working in weight management, I've never seen anyone successfully lose weight, and keep it off, all by him or herself. The support and encouragement from friends, family, co-workers, professionals and like-minded dieters is absolutely critical. As you make your way through losing weight, you'll need to cultivate a network of people and resources—and you'll call on them for different types of support at different times.

Take a few minutes to think about the kinds of support you need, then consider who might be able to give it to you. List as many people or sources as you can think of.

6 Strategies for Savvy Ordering in a Restaurant

* Read the whole menu. Get a feel for what's available and estimate the calories before you make a decision about what to order.

* Be the first to order. That way you won't be tempted to go along when the rest of the gang orders more than you'd like to eat.

* Consider à la carte. Try getting a soup or salad and an appetizer, or a couple of side dishes, instead of an overly large entree. Many restaurants these days offer smaller "tasting" plates or tapas-size portions too. They are worth a try and often just right in size.

* Split the difference. If an entrée sounds like too much food, see if one of your dining companions would like to share it with you. Or set aside half of the food as soon as it arrives and ask the waiter to wrap it up for you.

* Ask for sauces and dressings on the side. Most restaurants use a heavy hand with toppings; they just can't help themselves. When they're on the side you can control the amount without having to miss out. Rather than pouring them on, dip the tip of your fork into the dressing or sauce, then take a bite of food, so you'll get a little taste in every bite.

* Ask questions. Request that food be prepared your way, within reason (asking for a salad on the side instead of chips is reasonable; asking to have the fish and chips special steamed instead of fried is not). Ask politely but unapologetically; remember, restaurants are in the service business. Most are more than willing to accommodate your request—after all, you're paying!

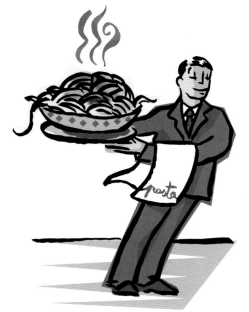

- **Emotional support:** People who can listen when you need someone to talk to, encourage you to keep going when you're feeling frustrated, and celebrate your successes. Possible sources: Your partner, relatives, friends, coworkers, fellow dieters, others.

Who can you call on?

_____

_____

_____

- **Practical support:** People to exercise and/or shop for healthy foods with, swap cooking ideas and recipes with, or even help with occasional child care or home chores so that you can still work out on extra-busy days. Possible sources: Your partner, relatives, friends, coworkers, fellow dieters, fellow activity or outdoor club members, others.

Who can you call on?

_____

_____

_____

- **Information:** Sources for answers about choosing healthy foods, exercising, staying emotionally healthy, general problem-solving. Possible sources: Health professionals (especially a registered dietitian), health organization websites, organized weight-loss groups, your local hospital's weight-management program, reputable books and magazines (see the "Resources" section, page 235).

Who can you call on, or where can you go?

_____

_____

_____

Once you've realized what you need and who can help you, start connecting the dots. Ask your designated supporter(s) if they're willing to help—and if so, talk about how they can support you—and be sure to thank them in advance.

If they're not willing or able to help, go back to the list of "possible sources" and think about how you can expand the list. Try connecting with someone else who's watching their weight—say, someone at work, at the health club or a parent at your child's school. Or try an organized online or in-person weight-loss support group that's associated with a hospital weight-loss clinic. You deserve to have a champion (or ten) in your corner!

DIET SABOTEURS

As powerful as it can be to have the support of your loved ones, it's equally frustrating if some of them seem to undermine your weight-loss efforts. It might be your Uncle Steve, who teases you for taking only a small portion of his "famous" lasagna. Or your spouse, who buys your favorite ice cream even though you're trying to keep temptations out of the house.

Many times, these so-called diet "saboteurs" really don't intend to do you harm. But deep down, some truly might not want you to lose weight. Consciously or unconsciously, friends might think that you're leaving them behind, especially if you both share a weight problem. Your spouse may worry that a slimmer you will attract competing attention from others. And any of them could fear that when you lose weight, you'll become a different person who might treat them differently too.

If you have reason to think that someone close to you is getting in the way of your weight-loss goals, don't wait to take action: talk about it. Without making any accusations, let them know how their actions affect you. Chances are, the saboteur is clueless; Uncle Steve honestly might not understand that "a little" lasagna makes a big dent in your daily calorie tally. Talk it over and work out a solution you can both live with.

But if you find your loved one truly isn't behind you, you'll need to look elsewhere for the support you need and deserve. Return to the facing page for more ideas.

> "I'm lucky that my husband is real supportive. He's a triathlete, so he's in amazing shape and has no body fat whatsoever—but he's never given me a hard time…I'm really appreciative, even though I can't keep up with him!"
> —**Susannah**, 49 (10 pounds lost)

NOW, YOU TRY IT: **CALL IN THE TROOPS**

The following are three scenarios that call for some support. Consult your list of support sources, then describe how you'd handle each one.

1) Your significant other is addicted to corn chips and noisily munches them while you're both watching TV. All you can think about is digging your hand into the bag too.

    Your plan:

    _____

    _____

2) You've had it. You're trying so hard to lose weight, but it seems like every day you "blow it" by missing a workout or giving in to a chocolate craving. You're ready to throw the scale out the window.

    Your plan:

    _____

    _____

3) You're confounded by the choices at the cafeteria. Are you better off with a chicken salad wrap or a grilled chicken sandwich?

    Your plan:

    _____

    _____

HOW TO BECOME A PROBLEM-SOLVER

Now that you have an appreciation for the problems that can come up as you move closer to your weight-loss goals, let's apply those skills to solving a specific problem that matters most to you. In general, problem-solving involves four steps:

1) **Identify the problem.**

2) **Generate a list of possible solutions.**

3) **Choose a solution.**

4) **Implement the plan.**

The best way to show how the problem-solving process works is to apply it to a familiar scenario: Let's say that every Sunday, your mother-in-law—we'll call her Zelda—makes a high-calorie brunch for the extended family, and your presence is, to put it mildly, required. You don't want to blow all your daily calories before noon, but if you decline what's being served, Zelda makes it clear that she feels insulted. Here's how you might tackle the problem.

1) Define the problem:

• Zelda feels hurt when someone doesn't eat her specialties; you want to please her.

• She doesn't offer any low-calorie options at her brunches.

• Other relatives who enjoy the meal encourage you to join in.

• Brunch is usually right after church, when you're hungry, which makes it harder for you to say no.

2) Generate possible solutions:

• You could refuse the invitation to brunch.

• You could discuss your concerns with Zelda and try to work out a compromise—say, offer to bring a low-calorie dish to complement her menu.

• You could eat a light snack before the brunch.

3) Choose a solution:

Select what seems to be the best solution; it doesn't have to be the perfect solution. Make as many people happy as you can, but be assertive about what you need too. There's no one "right" way to handle every problem, and what works in one situation might not work in another. For some, having a light snack beforehand to cut hunger might do the trick; others might feel it necessary to discuss the issue with Zelda, to give her a better understanding of the problem.

4) Implement the plan:

Take action as soon as you've chosen a solution—and later, assess its effectiveness. If it didn't work as well as you would have liked, don't worry. Many problems require multiple attempts before reaching resolution. Go back to the drawing board and try another strategy.

CHECK-IN: TACKLE A TRICKY PROBLEM

Think of a problem that challenges your weight-loss resolve. Then use your problem-solving skills to come up with possible solutions.

IDENTIFY THE PROBLEM.

_____

_____

_____

_____

GENERATE AT LEAST 3 POSSIBLE SOLUTIONS.

1. _____

2. _____

3. _____

_____

_____

PICK THE BEST SOLUTION.

_____

_____

HOW WILL YOU IMPLEMENT THE PLAN?

_____

_____

_____

CHAPTER 5

LIVING WELL

HAVING—AND KEEPING—THE BEST TOOLS TO MAKE YOUR WEIGHT LOSS A LIFE-LONG STRATEGY

You've been following your eating plan, sticking with your exercise goals. You're getting results. You are eating better foods and have found great new substitutions for the heavy fare of your past. You feel healthier and more energetic, and your clothes are looser. You might even be at your goal weight as you read this—terrific!

Now, for the hard part.

Believe it or not, you're entering the toughest phase of weight management. Diet experts call it "weight maintenance," but it may help just to think of it as "the rest of your life." For unlike following a weight-loss diet—which by definition has a beginning and an end—getting the pounds off is just one part of a lifelong strategy. Fortunately, you've already acquired the skills needed to stay on track, and as always, preparation and planning will see you through. You're ready for the last step of the process: creating a long-term strategy that will make your successes stick.

STEP 7: HAVE A LONG-TERM PLAN

You've come a long way in changing your behaviors, trading old, unhealthy habits for new ones. But it's important to understand that your old ways will come back to haunt you once in a while, and you will lapse. Maybe you'll eat too much at your niece's wedding. Or you'll sneak one of your friend's French fries while he's in the restroom, then realize you've finished them before he makes it back to the table. Lapses like these are normal! Don't beat yourself up over them.

The key is to get back on track, and quickly, when you lapse into old behaviors. The sooner you react, the easier it is to move on. If you don't react, you can easily slip back into an old behavior pattern, and your lapse becomes a relapse—or even a collapse if you give up altogether. As you move through these stages it becomes increasingly harder to recover, but it's never too late. You can always start over, though it will be harder the longer you've waited.

The first step in breaking the Lapse-Relapse-Collapse cycle is to understand how it works:

A **lapse** is a short-term slip-up in your routine that, if caught early, is easy to overcome. The eating binge at your niece's wedding is a good example: overindulging at a celebration won't derail your long-term goals, and you can easily nip it in the bud (see "How to Stop a Binge," page 76). If you eat a little less the next day or two to compensate, you'll likely be right back where you left off.

> "I always tell my wife, 'Carry 75 pounds around on your back and see what that feels like.' That's what it was like for me...I actually tried putting 50 pounds of weights in a backpack once and went for a walk. Boy, how did I carry that around for all those years?"
>
> —**John,** 50 (75 pounds lost)

> **"**There is no point at which you can say, 'Well, I'm successful now. I might as well take a nap.'**"**
>
> CARRIE FISHER, ACTRESS

A **relapse** is a breakdown in your ability to maintain a behavior change. You lapse, then lapse again, and gradually the old habits start creeping back. If you wake up the morning after the wedding and decide to load up at the breakfast buffet because you've "already blown it," that's a relapse.

A **collapse** is a complete breakdown of the behavior changes you've made: days after the wedding, you still find yourself overeating, and feeling like there's no turning back. Most people who have "collapsed" gain back the weight they've lost, and sometimes more.

It's clear that the critical step in this process comes right at the beginning, in how you handle a lapse. As always, planning makes a huge difference: defusing the lapse is much easier if you have a "back on track" strategy at the ready. Here are some ways successful weight maintainers handle lapses:

- Jim takes an extra-long walk the next day.

- Terry doesn't eat sweets or snacks for two or three days.

- Evan omits his daily glass of wine with dinner for a few days.

- Mona writes her feelings in a journal.

- Sandra weighs and measures her food portions until she feels back in control.

- Jeff calls his exercise buddy for a pep talk.

> **You must have long-term goals to keep you from being frustrated by short-term failures.**
>
> CHARLES C. NOBLE

RAISE THE RED FLAG ON LAPSES

Everyone has lapses—but what's the difference between those who can recover, and who can't? When researchers looked at the successful weight losers in the National Weight Control Registry, and compared them to some who'd regained back some of their weight after one or two years, they found that even a small weight gain

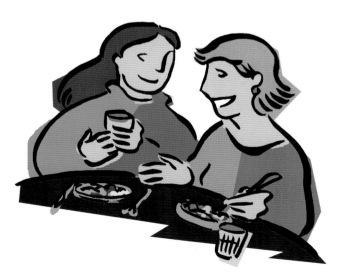

was hard to reverse: those who'd regained the most weight were the least likely to be able to take it off again. That's extra incentive for you to act quickly on a relapse—and also to keep weighing yourself regularly. (If you can't seem to face the scale and have stopped weighing yourself, it's time to do something. First get on the scale and confront the reality. Start weighing yourself every day, at the same time. A growing body of research supports daily weigh-ins as a method to avoid weight gain or regain.)

It's a good idea to designate a "red flag" weight—say, 3 to 5 pounds above your weight goal. If you see that weight on the scale, consider it a signal that you need to act immediately with a "back on track" strategy.

THE 6-STEP PLAN FOR RELAPSE PREVENTION

1) Step back and ask, "What happened?" Look objectively at what brought on the lapse.

2) Calm down. Take a few deep breaths and remind yourself, "One slip-up does not make me a failure."

3) Renew your vows. Remind yourself of how far you have come, and how disappointed you'll be if this one slip-up undoes all your hard work.

4) Learn from it. Think about what pushed you to your lapse (your food diary notes can help). What can you do differently next time?

5) Implement your "back on track" strategy right away.

6) Call for backup. Ask for help from those people who are supportive and who want you to succeed (*see "Call in the Troops," page 71*).

How to Stop a Binge

When you feel a colossal eating episode coming on, ask yourself:

1. Am I truly hungry? If you're not sure, wait 20 minutes, then ask yourself again.

2. Has it been 3 hours since I last ate? (If not, your hunger may be more emotional than physical).

3. Can a small snack, like a handful of carrots or grapes and a few peanuts, tide me over until the next meal?

Score one for daily weighing

If you're not weighing yourself every day, maybe it's time to start. New support for daily weighing comes from the STOPRegain trial, led by Rena Wing, director of The Weight Control and Diabetes Research Center at the Miriam Hospital in Providence, where the National Weight Control Registry is based.

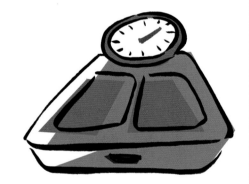

Recently, Wing and her colleagues looked at the weight-maintenance strategies of 314 people who'd lost an average of 44 pounds. The "losers" used one of three methods to help them prevent regaining: regular face-to-face counseling, an Internet weight-loss program or weight-loss-focused newsletters. More people in the face-to-face and Internet groups weighed themselves daily (71 percent and 65.2 percent, respectively), while less than a third of the newsletter readers did.

After 18 months, weight regain was the smallest in the face-to-face group—only 2.5 pounds—and the Internet group (6 pounds). By contrast, the newsletter group—the ones who largely eschewed daily weighing—had gained back an average of more than 10 pounds!

NOW, YOU TRY IT:

YOUR BACK-ON-TRACK STRATEGIES

Describe a lapse or relapse that you've experienced with weight management.

_____

_____

_____

In retrospect, what could you have done differently in that situation?

_____

_____

_____

Spell out at least two "back-on-track" strategies for the next time you have a lapse or relapse.

_____

_____

_____

_____

THE ALL-OR-NOTHING-THINKING TRAP

One of the reasons a lapse can so quickly become a relapse is the tendency many of us have to think in black-and-white extremes: chocolate is bad, carrots are good; one slip-up means you've fallen off the wagon. Cognitive therapists call this distorted thought pattern "all or nothing" thinking, and ultimately it can harm your efforts to lose weight. Here are some symptoms:

- Outlawing "bad" foods. Sometimes you're tempted by a food simply because you've sworn off it as "forbidden." And if you can't resist taking a bite, it's easy to slide into all-out breakdown: "I've blown it by eating two cookies. I might as well finish the whole bag."

- Using words like "always," "must" or "never." Imperatives like these set impossible standards—and set you up for feeling like a failure when you (inevitably) don't live up to them. You can't "always" avoid sweets or "never" eat French fries again. Likewise, saying you "must" walk 10,000 steps every day means that when something thwarts your plan—say, an emergency project at work—you might be tempted to give up altogether.

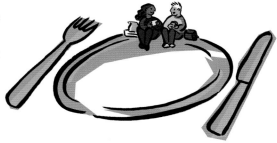

The best way to avoid these traps is to recognize when you're falling into them. Hearing yourself say words like "must" or "never" is a big clue; listen for these words when you're talking, and make a conscious effort to replace them with more flexible words, like "sometimes." The more you practice, the easier it will be. Here's how you might rewrite the script:

ALL-OR-NOTHING THOUGHT:	COUNTER THOUGHT:
I will never eat pizza again.	I'll try to choose alternatives to pizza most of the time, but when I do have some, I'll have just one slice, and enjoy it.
I must take a daily 2-mile walk.	I'll try to take a walk every day, but if something prevents me from walking I'll try to jump rope, or do calisthenics while I watch TV.
I'm never going to be an exerciser.	I haven't exercised much in the past, but if I try to get moving most days and keep looking for new activities, it will become easier and more fun.

DON'T BEAT YOURSELF UP

As you're moving toward your goals, how do you encourage yourself? Are you a "cheerleader" who treats yourself with love and kindness, celebrating your successes and acknowledging your slip-ups with forgiveness and empathy? Or are you the "bad coach," who prods with negative thoughts like "What a loser!" and berates you anytime you don't perform perfectly?

Your internal thoughts about yourself and your abilities can have a huge impact on your progress. If you treat yourself like a failure, it can become a self-fulfilling prophecy. Without the support of your most important champion—yourself—it's easy to feel demoralized. And that might just move you to give up trying. After all, if you're truly that hopeless, why bother to change?

Think of how you might offer positive words of encouragement to someone else and then use the same approach on yourself. It can, and does, work.

If you work to replace negative internal thoughts with positive ones, you can turn a minor setback into a small victory. For example, instead of gnashing your teeth over those two pounds you gained, focus on the 10 pounds you've already lost, and learn from the experience: "I gained two pounds this week, but my net loss is still eight pounds. And after all, it was a stressful week at work. Next time, I'll hit the gym rather than the cookies."

> "[My VTrim leader] always said, 'Just write down what you eat. Don't pass judgment on it, just treat it as data. Look at the data, and treat it as data.'"
> —Julie, 47 (45 pounds lost)

> You wouldn't urge your friend to "move it, blubberbutt!" So why would you use that language to chide yourself? Treat yourself with kindness and with an upbeat attitude—like a friend—and you'll have a much better chance of success.

To put a positive spin on a negative thought, you'll need to:
- Be conscious of potential problems.
- Identify the negative thoughts, training yourself to listen for them.
- Counter the negative thoughts with positive counter thoughts.

Here are a few examples of how this process works:

POTENTIAL PROBLEM: BURNOUT.

Negative Thought:

"I've been on this program for weeks, and I still have a lot of weight to lose. If I don't see some big results soon, I'm going to quit."

Counter Thought:

"I know that effective weight loss isn't easy, and it isn't fast. It took a long time for me to gain this weight, and it will take me a while to lose it. But if I quit now, I erase all the progress I've made. If I've lasted this long, I can stick with it!"

POTENTIAL PROBLEM: SELF-CRITICISM.

Negative Thought:

"If I've lost weight, why do I still look huge in these pants?"

Counter Thought:

"I still have some distance to go, but already my pants are feeling looser. And I don't get out of breath when I walk up the hill to my office anymore. I'm making progress both inside and out."

> **"We're all in this alone."**
>
> LILY TOMLIN, COMEDIAN

PARTING WORDS: GO THE DISTANCE!

However far you've come on your weight-loss journey, you have plenty to celebrate. Just making one behavioral change takes lots of work and planning, and you've tackled many. You've made plans and put them into action—and anticipated and planned for the inevitable, occasional setback. You've already shown that you have what it takes to maintain this new, healthier lifestyle you've chosen for yourself.

And, while you might be nervous that you're going to become one of those many people who regains the lost weight in short order, there are plenty of reasons why you won't go that way. Here are just a few:

- You've done your homework. You've assessed whether you're ready for change, and set realistic short- and long-term goals for yourself.

- You've mastered the essential tools that successful weight losers rely on. Self-tracking your eating and activity patterns, and weighing yourself regularly will keep you on track for life.

- You've become someone who eats less and moves more. And along the way, you've learned lifelong skills for shopping, cooking and ordering healthy meals and for building and supporting a regular exercise habit.

- You've become a problem solver. You've figured out how to keep your eating and exercise goals in sight, despite the unexpected. You've made fall-back plans and default restaurant menu orders, and even learned how to handle saboteurs.

> "My kids have been so supportive. They've said, 'Mom, we love you however you are, but you seem a lot happier being a bit on the thinner side.'"
>
> —**Gail,** 53 (50 pounds lost)

- You've learned how to identify problem behaviors and negative thinking, and replace them with healthy attitudes and habits.

- You know where to turn for support. You've identified the people and resources in your life that you can call on whenever you need information, direction, inspiration or just a listening ear.

Look back in your food diaries and activity logs, and you'll see that you've accomplished a major turn-around in your thinking and your actions. As your journey continues, you'll keep revising and changing your goals, and I expect you'll come back to these pages regularly to refresh your skills. You can also use the next chapter's menus and planning tips for a fresh start anytime, or whenever you need inspiration. And, with the wonderful recipes that follow—which you'll turn to time and again—we have the makings of a promising lifetime partnership.

Finally, it will pay to remember that weight loss is not the ultimate goal of all you have done and are committed to doing.

Losing pounds, for the many, many thousands who have done it before you, is the door opener to a new life—one with more energy, more vitality and more self-confidence. It is often a precursor to healthier relationships with family, friends and significant others. It can be the key to being able to do new and exciting things—professionally and personally—that you previously avoided.

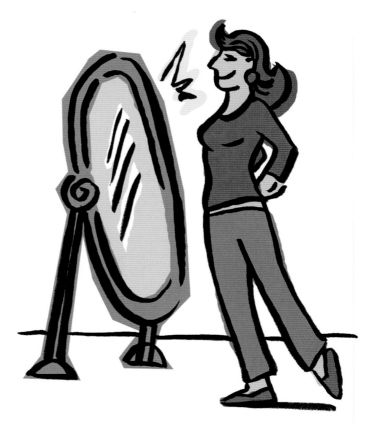

❝ It's not that I'm so smart, it's just that I stay with problems longer. ❞

ALBERT EINSTEIN

❝ Being defeated is often a temporary condition. Giving up is what makes it permanent. ❞

MARILYN VOS SAVANT,
COLUMNIST & AUTHOR

Getting rid of excess weight is much more than leaving behind physical mass—it lightens your whole emotional load in ways that you may not even have envisioned. The behavioral tools and new habits you've developed will serve to not just keep the scales under control, but also as instruments for helping tune a more harmonious way of life for many years to come. Losing weight is not, of course, a panacea, but for many people, the ongoing sense of empowerment at using their own wits and willpower to look and feel better becomes a cornerstone of their lives.

Here's to your success, now and always!

NOW, YOU TRY IT: REWRITE YOUR SCRIPT

Think of three bumps in the road that may get in the way of your weight loss. Now, transform the negative attitudes you anticipate into positive, affirming statements.

1. Potential Problem:

_____

_____

Negative Thought:

_____

_____

Counter Thought:

_____

_____

_____

2. Potential Problem:

_____

_____

Negative Thought:

_____

_____

Counter Thought:

_____

_____

_____

3. Potential Problem:

_____

_____

Negative Thought:

_____

_____

Counter Thought:

_____

_____

_____

CHECK-IN: YOUR LONG-TERM SUCCESS PLAN

Take a long look back at the work you've done and how far you've come. Then, lay the groundwork for the future, by reviewing your most important assets and achievements.

Repeat this exercise or revisit this page every few months or so, revising it if you need to. That way you'll always keep your weight-management goals in focus.

1) Which behavior change was most helpful to you for losing weight, and why? Think of the steps you've taken—keeping a food diary and activity log, planning meals, identifying and calling on your supporters, and more.

_____

_____

_____

_____

_____

2) How will you handle the following unexpected setbacks?
a) You planned a long workout, but your in-laws drop by for a surprise visit. What do you do?

_____

_____

_____

_____

b) You ordered a single portion of "Garden Pasta," but the waiter brings you something you never expected: a manhole-cover-sized platter of pasta drenched in cheesy sauce, with just a few scattered bits of vegetables. What do you do? What will you do next time you order something you've never ordered before?

_____

_____

_____

_____

3) You're feeling very stressed out. What will you do?

_____

_____

And if that doesn't work?

_____

_____

And then?

_____

_____

4) Name four people who will help when you need them. Define each person's specific role.

WHO? _____

HOW WILL HE/SHE HELP? _____

_____

_____

WHO? _____

HOW WILL HE/SHE HELP? _____

_____

_____

WHO? _____

HOW WILL HE/SHE HELP? _____

_____

_____

WHO? _____

HOW WILL HE/SHE HELP? _____

_____

_____

CHAPTER 6

WHAT TO EAT?

28 DAYS TO A NEW, LEANER LIFE

You've read the chapters, you've grasped the guidelines, you have the materials you need to track your progress, you've done your planning, you've lined up your supporters and you've set your goals. Now you're ready to go and blaze your own path.

But you may still be asking, "What can I eat?"

Perhaps you need ideas for dinner tonight—or what to pack for lunches this week, since you've made "brown-bagging-it" one of your weight-loss strategies. Or perhaps you just need a little push to get started in the right direction of planning, shopping and cooking healthful meals. This chapter is where you bring everything to the table and see how it looks and tastes.

The EATINGWELL Mix & Match Menus were developed to inspire newcomers to our weight-loss program—or to help recharge you anytime you need to come back for a boost. You'll find sound ideas from EATINGWELL's Test Kitchen and recipe wizards for four weeks of great eating. The breakfast, lunch, dinner and snack menus are all designed by our nutrition editors to be interchangeable, so switch them around as you please. If you like, eat the same meal for breakfast every day, or choose only vegetarian options one week; as long as you keep the meals in the same categories (exchanging, say, only lunches for lunches) you'll be getting a well-balanced, varied and creative menu, and we've done the calorie-counting for you.

The menus provide approximately 1,500 calories per day, with room for adjusting if your calorie goals are higher or lower. We've estimated the calories for each day's menu conservatively, allowing you a little "wiggle room," since experience with food records shows that most people eat more than they estimate.

> ### The EATINGWELL Formula
>
> Recipes and menus presented in this volume fit the basic 1,500-calorie-per-day guidelines for the EATINGWELL Diet:
>
> - Breakfasts at about 350 calories.
> - Lunches at about 500 calories.
> - Dinners at about 500 calories.
> - Snacks or discretionary drinks at about 150 calories.
>
> If your calorie goals are above or below 1,500 calories, you can adjust portion sizes, add or subtract side dishes and "extras" (dessert, beverages) as needed.

No matter which menus you choose, you'll be eating well, with an abundance of whole-grains to provide extra fiber and micronutrients that help you feel and stay fuller, longer. Lunches and dinners feature ample servings of a colorful variety of vegetables, and you'll get at least two daily servings of fruit. There are three daily servings of low-fat dairy foods to meet your calcium needs, along with high-quality protein and vitamins A and D. If you can't tolerate or prefer not to choose dairy products, we recommend substituting low-fat or fat-free soy milk products. Read the labels carefully to make sure they are fortified with vitamins A and D, and look for brands that have minimal or no added sugars.

We've planned for the occasional restaurant meals and brown-bagged lunches, the occasional glass of wine or beer, and even a few grand-occasion splurges. Best of all, we've kept the preparation fast and simple, so you can spend less time in the kitchen.

The next 28 days can be among the most important of your life, as you begin your journey to a new relationship with food. Studies show it takes a good while for behavior changes to take hold and become new habits. Some of our VTrim program participants report that their newer, healthier lifestyle already starts to feel like a routine by as early as three weeks to a month, while it takes others several months.

These menus will give you what you need to get in the habit of cooking and meal planning that fits with your weight-loss goals. Plug yourself into them today, and by the end of four weeks you'll be well on your way to having a priceless set of new, healthy habits. And you'll have eaten abundantly and perhaps better than you have in years.

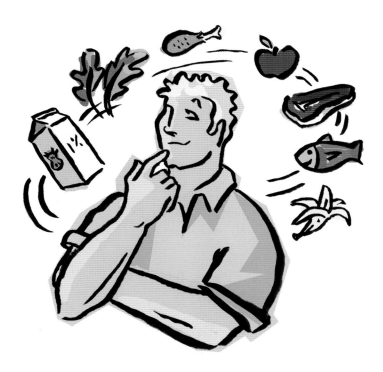

MEAL/ COURSE	Day 1	CALORIES	Day 2	CALORIES	Day 3	CALORIES	Day 4	CALORIES
Breakfast	Quick Breakfast Taco (p. 107)	123	Tomato & Ham Breakfast Melt (p. 107)	299	EW Diet Breakfast Smoothie (p. 106)	355	Spinach & Tomato Omelet (p. 100)	152
	Skim milk (1 cup) or nonfat plain yogurt (6 oz.)	95	Tomato juice (1 cup)	50			Skim milk (1 cup)	83
	Orange (1 medium)	62					Berries or melon (1 cup)	60
Lunch	The EatingWell Cobb Salad (p. 111)	314	Crackers & Tuna (p. 203)	229	Romaine Salad with Orange, Feta & Beans (p. 114)	242	The EatingWell Tuna Melt (p. 202)	264
	Whole-wheat toast (1 slice)	69	EW Diet House Salad (p. 121)	71	Whole-wheat pita bread (½)	85	EW Diet House Salad (p. 121)	71
	Low-fat cheese (1 ½ oz.)	95	Banana (6-inch)	90	Hummus & Vegetables (p. 230)	108	Skim milk (1 cup) or nonfat plain yogurt (6 oz.)	95
Snack	Hummus & Vegetables (p. 230)	108	Low-fat vanilla yogurt (6 oz.)	145	Ham & Pepper Rollups (p. 230)	100	Cereal Mix (p. 229)	124
Dinner: *Main Dish*	Almond-Crusted Chicken Fingers (p. 162)	175	Crab Cake Burgers (p. 201)	161	Spicy Beef with Shrimp & Bok Choy (p. 214)	204	Curried Chicken with Mango Salad (p. 173)	289
Side	Whole-wheat couscous (½ cup) (p. 228)	140	Skim milk (1 cup) or low-fat cheese (1 ½ oz.)	95	Brown Rice & Greens (p. 222)	113	Quick-cooking barley (½ cup) (p. 228)	86
Vegetable	Mary's Zucchini (p. 223)	83	Oven Sweet Potato Fries (p. 222)	122				
Salad	Cucumber Salad (p. 122)	24	Lemony Carrot Salad (p. 122)	90	Napa Cabbage Slaw (p. 122)	93	EW Diet House Salad (p. 121)	71
Dessert or Drink	Cinnamon Baked Apples (p. 232)	138	Berries or melon (1 cup)	60	Broiled Mango (p. 232)	69	Sorbet Shake (p. 231)	172
TOTAL DAILY CALORIES		1,426		1,412		1,369		1,467

	CALORIES		CALORIES		CALORIES
Day 5		**Day 6**		**Day 7**	
Cheddar-Apple Melt (p. 106)	253	Asparagus & Canadian Bacon Omelet (p. 98)	198	Herb & Onion Frittata (p. 99)	192
Skim milk (1 cup) *or* nonfat plain yogurt (6 oz.)	95	Skim milk (1 cup) *or* nonfat plain yogurt (6 oz.)	95	Skim milk (1 cup) *or* nonfat plain yogurt (6 oz.)	95
		Dried apricots (2)	34	Berries or melon (1 cup)	60
Loaded Spinach Salad (p. 110)	300	Ultimate Beef Chili (leftovers) (p. 216)	241	EatingWell Power Salad (p. 113)	180
Whole-wheat pita bread (½)	85	Rainbow Chopped Salad (p. 123)	64	Zucchini & Cheddar Soup (p. 139)	115
Low-fat cheese stick	100	Garlic-Tomato Toasts (p. 222)	91	Whole-wheat toast with melted Parmesan	115
Radish Crispbread (p. 231)	104	Cheesy Popcorn (p. 229)	75	Almonds (1 oz.)	169
				Apple (1 small)	62
Ultimate Beef Chili (p. 216)	241	Ham-&-Cheese-Stuffed Chicken Breasts (p. 163)	236	London Broil with Cherry-Balsamic Sauce (p. 210)	216
Whole-wheat toast (1 slice)	69	Provençal Barley (p. 222)	115	Buttermilk-Herb Mashed Potatoes (p. 222)	85
		Orange-Infused Green & Red Peppers (p. 223)	78	Wilted Spinach with Garlic (p. 224)	59
EW Diet House Salad (p. 121), Creamy Dill Ranch (p. 126)	53	EW Diet House Salad (p. 121)	71	Watercress Salad (p. 123)	38
Cinnamon Oranges (p. 233)	86	Grilled Peach Sundae (p. 233)	154	Broiled Mango (p. 232)	69
	1,386		**1,452**		**1,455**

WEEK 1

Calorie Goal: _____

Exercise Goal: _____

Notes:

_____

_____

_____

_____

_____

_____

_____

_____

_____

_____

_____

THIS WEEK:

Focus on getting used to writing down everything you eat and drink. Take your food diary with you everywhere, so that you can "write it after you bite it." Don't stress about doing it perfectly, but on just doing it. It will become much easier over time.

MEAL/ COURSE	Day 8	CALORIES	Day 9	CALORIES	Day 10	CALORIES	Day 11	CALORIES
Breakfast	Banana-Cocoa Soy Smoothie (p.106)	340	Breakfast Parfait (with cottage cheese) (p.106)	248	Raisin Bread & Farmer's Cheese (p.107)	243	Peanut Butter-Cinnamon English Muffin (p.106)	247
			Low-fat vanilla yogurt (6 oz.)	145	Grapefruit (½)	32	Skim milk (1 cup) or nonfat plain yogurt (6 oz.)	95
	Morning Snack: Gorp (p.229)	102			Skim milk (1 cup) or nonfat plain yogurt (6 oz.)	95		
Lunch	Roasted Tomato Soup (p.131)	95	Tuscan-Style Tuna Salad (p.203)	253	Chicken Noodle Soup with Dill (p.130)	191	Roasted Red Pepper Subs (p.146)	221
	Seared Chicken Salad with Edamame & Cilantro (p.116)	233	Whole-wheat pita bread (½)	85	Whole-wheat toast with melted low-fat cheese (1 oz.)	135	Zucchini & Cheddar Soup (p.139)	115
	Wasa cracker	30	Honeydew melon (1 cup)	61	EW Diet House Salad (p.121)	71	Banana (6-inch)	90
Snack	Cheesy Popcorn (p.229)	75	Fig Newmans (2)	120	Turkey Rollups (p.231)	82	Pickled Beets & Cheese (p.230) 2 Wasa crackers	85 60
Dinner: *Main Dish*	Sautéed Flounder with Orange-Shallot Sauce (p.191)	222	Florentine Ravioli (p.158)	277	Shrimp Caesar Salad (p.118)	339	EATINGWELL's Oven-Fried Chicken (p.164)	227
Side	Brown rice (½ cup) (p.228)	109			Wasa crackers (2)	60	Oven Fries (p.222)	103
Vegetable	Steamed broccoli (1 cup) (p.225)	20	Steamed cauliflower florets (1 cup) (p.226)	56			Carrot & celery sticks (½ cup)	20
Salad	Basic Green Salad with Vinaigrette (p.121)	115	Sliced Tomato Salad (p.123)	44			EW Diet House Salad (p.121), Blue Cheese Dressing (p.127)	72
Dessert or Drink	Banana-Cinnamon Frozen Yogurt (p.232)	126	Raspberry-Mango Sundae (p.234)	167	Banana-Cinnamon Frozen Yogurt (p.232)	126	Tea-Scented Mandarins (p.234)	63
TOTAL DAILY CALORIES		**1,467**		**1,456**		**1,374**		**1,398**

Day 12		Day 13		Day 14	
Cereal (dry, 1 cup)	120	Oatmeal (cooked, 1 cup)	148	Ham, Gruyère & Spinach Bread Pudding (p. 101)	276
Banana (6-inch)	90	Berries or melon (1 cup)	60	Apple (1 small, sliced)	62
Skim milk (1 cup)	83	Skim milk (1 cup) or nonfat plain yogurt (6 oz.)	95		
Loaded Spinach Salad (p. 110)	300	Spicy Vegetable Soup (p. 133)	253	EATINGWELL Power Salad (p. 113)	180
Oatmeal bread (1 slice)	73	Whole-wheat toast with melted low-fat Swiss cheese (1 oz.)	168	Whole-wheat breadsticks (1 oz.)	100
Cottage cheese (1/2 cup)	90			Berries or melon (1 cup)	60
Shrimp Cocktail (p. 231)	74	Pears & Blue Cheese (p. 230)	96	Cajun Spiced Hard-Boiled Egg (p. 229)	68
Turkey-Mushroom Burger (p. 182)	193	Herb & Lemon Roast Chicken (p. 170)	157	Coffee-Braised Pot Roast with Caramelized Onions (p. 208)	252
Whole-wheat English muffin	134	Roasted new potatoes (1 cup) (p. 226)	220	Roasted new potatoes (1/2 cup) (p. 226)	110
Tomato slice and lettuce (on burger)	15	Zucchini & Mushroom Sauté (p. 224)	37	Steamed cauliflower florets (1 cup) (p. 226)	50
Rainbow Chopped Salad (p. 123)	64	The Wedge (p. 123)	70	EW Diet House Salad (p. 121)	71
Sorbet Shake (p. 231)	172	Grilled Peach Sundae (p. 233)	154	Pineapple-Coconut Frappe (p. 234)	143
	1,408		**1,458**		**1,378**

WEEK 2

Calorie Goal: _____
Exercise Goal: _____

Notes:

_____
_____
_____
_____
_____
_____
_____
_____
_____
_____
_____
_____

THIS WEEK:

Feeling hungry? Make sure you don't go more than five hours without eating, so your appetite stays on an even keel. Include a little protein at every meal and snack, and concentrate on getting at least three daily servings of whole grains. (Use the "Key Foods Checklist" in your food diary to help you keep track.)

MEAL/ COURSE	Day 15	CALORIES	Day 16	CALORIES	Day 17	CALORIES	Day 18	CALORIES
Breakfast	EW Diet Breakfast Smoothie (p. 106)	355	Oatmeal (cooked, 1 cup)	148	Blueberry-Coconut-Macadamia Muffin (p. 103)	202	Oatmeal (cooked, 1 cup)	148
			Skim milk (1 cup) or nonfat plain yogurt (6 oz.)	95	Skim milk (1 cup) or nonfat plain yogurt (6 oz.)	95	Nonfat plain yogurt (6 oz.)	95
	Morning Snack: Gorp (p. 229)	102	Banana (6-inch)	90	Apple (1 small, sliced)	62	Honeydew melon (1 cup)	61
Lunch	Egg Salad Sandwich with Watercress (p. 148)	289	Butter-Bean Spread Roll-Up Sandwich (p. 147)	343	Tuscan-Style Tuna Salad (p. 203)	253	Shrimp Louis Salad Sandwich (p. 200)	210
	Chickpea Salad (p. 122)	90	Cajun Spice Hard-Boiled Egg (p. 229)	68	Low-fat cheese stick	100	Carrot sticks (½ cup), Creamy Ranch Dressing (2 Tbsp.) (p. 126)	45
	Skim milk (1 cup) or nonfat plain yogurt (6 oz.)	95					Skim milk (1 cup) or nonfat plain yogurt (6 oz.)	95
Snack	Ham & Pepper Rollups (p. 230)	100	Tamari almonds (1 oz.)	169	Cucumbers & Cottage Cheese (p. 229)	104	Butter-Bean Spread & Rice Cakes (p. 229)	60
Dinner: Main Dish	Warm Salmon Salad with Crispy Potatoes (p. 120)	262	Chicken with Creamy Chive Sauce (p. 175)	248	Mediterranean Portobello Burger (p. 142)	301	Marmalade Chicken (p. 174)	213
Side			Buttermilk-Herb Mashed Potatoes (p. 222)	85			Brown rice (½ cup) (p. 228)	109
Vegetable	Lemony Carrot Salad (p. 122)	90	Steamed asparagus (½ cup) (p. 225)	23	Trio of Peas (p. 224)	74	Wilted Spinach with Garlic (p. 224)	59
Salad			Basic Green Salad with Vinaigrette (p. 121)	115	Chopped Tomato Salad (p. 122)	65	EW Diet House Salad (p. 121)	71
Dessert or Drink	Fresh fruit (1 cup)	60	Honeydew melon (1 cup)	61	Chocolate Malted Ricotta (p. 232)	152	Choice of dessert	250
TOTAL DAILY CALORIES		**1,443**		**1,445**		**1,408**		**1,416**

	CALORIES		CALORIES		CALORIES
Day 19		**Day 20**		**Day 21**	
Blueberry-Coconut-Macadamia Muffin (p. 103)	202	Peanut Butter-Cinnamon English Muffin (p. 106)	247	EW Diet Breakfast Smoothie (p. 106)	355
Skim milk (1 cup) *or* nonfat plain yogurt (6 oz.)	95	Skim milk (1 cup) *or* nonfat plain yogurt (6 oz.)	95		
Apple (1 small, sliced)	62				
Curried Tofu Salad (p. 156)	140	Romaine Salad with Orange, Feta & Beans (p. 114)	242	Italian Peasant Soup with Cabbage, Beans & Cheese (p. 135)	303
Whole-wheat pita bread (½)	85	Garlic-Tomato Toasts (p. 222)	91	Whole-wheat toast with melted low-fat cheese (1 oz.)	135
Tomato slice and lettuce (on sandwich)	15				
Sorbet Shake (p. 231)	172	The Perfect Snack (p. 230)	123	Guacamole-Stuffed Eggs (p. 230)	55
Chili-Rubbed Tilapia with Asparagus & Lemon (p. 194)	210	Chicken with Green Olives & Prunes (p. 177)	224	Southwestern Steak & Peppers (p. 209)	231
Brown rice (½ cup) (p. 228)	109	Whole-wheat couscous (½ cup) (p. 228)	140	Roasted sweet potato (½ cup) (p. 227)	122
Cucumber Salad (p. 122)	24	Steamed broccoli (1 cup) (p. 225)	20		
EW Diet House Salad (p. 121)	71	Chickpea Salad (p. 122)	90	Rainbow Chopped Salad (p. 123)	64
Quick Cheesecake (p. 234)	239	Chocolate Malted Ricotta (p. 232)	152	Gingered Peach Gratin (p. 233)	168
	1,424		**1,424**		**1,433**

Calorie Goal: _____

Exercise Goal: _____

Notes:

_____

_____

_____

_____

_____

_____

_____

_____

_____

_____

_____

_____

_____

THIS WEEK:

If you haven't done it already, consider adding strength training to your exercise schedule. Most aerobic exercises, like walking, running, stair climbing or jumping rope, work the large muscles of the legs, but they don't do much for your arms and upper torso. Working those muscles will help you stand straighter, move and lift things more easily—and boost your calorie-burning rate.

MEAL/ COURSE	Day 22	CALORIES	Day 23	CALORIES	Day 24	CALORIES	Day 25	CALORIES
Breakfast	Asparagus & Canadian Bacon Omelet (p. 98)	198	Breakfast Parfait (with yogurt) (p. 106)	185	Raisin Bread & Farmer's Cheese (p. 107)	243	EW Diet Breakfast Smoothie (p. 106)	355
	Skim milk (1 cup) or nonfat plain yogurt (6 oz.)	95	Bagel (½) & low-fat cream cheese (1 Tbsp.)	108	Grapefruit (½)	32		
	Grapefruit (½)	32						
Lunch	Shrimp Caesar Salad (p. 118)	339	Creamy Tarragon Chicken Salad (p. 171)	227	Roasted Tomato Soup (p. 131)	95	The EATINGWELL Cobb Salad (p. 111)	314
	Whole-wheat Saltine crackers (6)	77	Whole-wheat pita bread (½)	85	Whole-grain toast, sliced turkey (1 oz.), part-skim Swiss cheese (1 oz.)	204	Whole-wheat Saltine crackers (6)	77
	Skim milk (1 cup) or nonfat plain yogurt (6 oz.)	95	Skim milk (1 cup) or nonfat plain yogurt (6 oz.)	95	Skim milk (1 cup) or nonfat plain yogurt (6 oz.)	95		
Snack	Eggcetera (p. 229)	88	Sesame Carrots (p. 231)	33	Gorp (p. 229)	102	Hummus & Vegetables (p. 230)	108
			Almonds (1 oz.)	169				
Dinner: *Main Dish*	Peanut-Ginger Tofu & Vegetables (p. 154)	221	Warm Salad of Greens, Italian Sausage & Potatoes (p. 119)	262	Mustard-Crusted Salmon (p. 190)	290	Spicy Chicken Tacos (p. 167)	303
Side	Brown rice (½ cup) (p. 228)	109	Garlic-Tomato Toasts (p. 222)	91	Brown rice (½ cup) (p. 228)	109	Vinegary Coleslaw (p. 123)	101
Vegetable	Sesame Green Beans (p. 224)	67	Roasted squash (½ cup) (p. 227)	83	Steamed asparagus (½ cup) (p. 225)	23		
Salad	EW Diet House Salad (p. 121)	71			EW Diet House Salad (p. 121), Orange-Oregano Dressing	61		
Dessert or Drink	Nectarine (1 medium)	60	Strawberries Dipped in Chocolate (p. 234)	49	Pineapple-Coconut Frappe (p. 234)	143	Spiced Hot Chocolate (p. 234)	175
TOTAL DAILY CALORIES		**1,447**		**1,387**		**1,397**		**1,433**

	CALORIES		CALORIES		CALORIES
Day 26		**Day 27**		**Day 28**	
Quick Breakfast Taco (p. 107)	123	Herb & Onion Frittata (p. 99)	192	Tomato & Ham Breakfast Melt (p. 107)	299
Skim milk (1 cup) *or* nonfat plain yogurt (6 oz.)	95	Skim milk (1 cup) *or* nonfat plain yogurt (6 oz.)	95	Grapefruit (½)	32
Banana (6-inch)	90	Berries *or* melon (1 cup)	60		
Egg Salad Sandwich with Watercress (p. 148)	289	Chicken Tortilla Soup (p. 137)	357	EATINGWELL Power Salad (p. 113)	180
Berries or melon (1 cup)	60	Grilled corn tortilla with low-fat Cheddar (1 oz.)	106	Low-fat vanilla yogurt (6 oz.)	145
Skim milk (1 cup) *or* nonfat plain yogurt (6 oz.)	95	EW Diet House Salad (p. 121)	71		
Pickled Beets & Cheese (p. 230)	85	Avocado Tea Sandwich (p. 229)	143	Almonds (1 oz.)	169
2 Wasa crackers	60				
Shrimp with Broccoli (p. 197)	178	Grilled Pork Tenderloin with Mustard, Rosemary & Apple Marinade (p. 219)	165	Golden Polenta & Egg with Mustard Sauce (p. 149)	287
Brown rice (½ cup) (p. 228)	109	Buttermilk-Herb Mashed Potatoes (p. 222)	85		
Wilted Spinach with Garlic (p. 224)	59	Warm Apple-Cabbage Slaw (p. 123)	68	Roasted squash (½ cup) (p. 227)	83
				Greens with Parmesan Vinaigrette (p. 122)	154
Gorp (p. 229)	102	Balsamic Vinegar-Spiked Strawberries (p. 232)	40	Frosted Grapes (p. 233)	55
	1,396		**1,382**		**1,404**

THIS WEEK:

Take stock. Look at your food diary and activity log from your first week, and note how far you've come. Don't just count miles walked or calories burned, but how you're feeling. Do you have more energy or are you sleeping better at night? And remember to reward yourself for the milestones you've reached and set new short-term goals.

CHAPTER 7

EAT WELL BY COOKING WELL

DELICIOUSLY SATISFYING, HEALTHY-IN-A-HURRY RECIPES FOR ALL MEALS AND OCCASIONS

While there is no shortage of smoking guns when investigators look at the rise in weight problems in this country, one key culprit is that we're preparing fewer and fewer of our own meals.

In recent years, the percentage of meals Americans eat "outside the home," whether restaurant or takeout fare, has grown at a rampant pace. And so have our waistlines; just chart the increase in obesity in the last few decades against the number of restaurant meals eaten in an average week, and you find obvious parallels. One recent study found that people who reported frequently eating breakfast or dinner at restaurants approximately doubled their risk of being obese.

To maximize sales, the restaurant trade has zeroed in on the flavor and texture sensations humans crave: creamy, crispy, salty, sweet. Many eateries have cranked up the levels of fats, sugars, and sodium in everything they serve, while mega-sizing portions. Wash it all down with millions of servings of soft drinks, and you have a recipe for an obesity epidemic.

Eating and cooking at home, it turns out, may be one of the best tactics you can use for losing weight and maintaining a well-earned weight loss. When you do the cooking, you have hands-on control of all the ingredients, cooking methods and portion sizes. With the right recipes, you can even serve up foods with all the flavors and sensory pleasures you crave, but with only a fraction of the calories, saturated fat and sodium.

Thankfully, it's easy to do your own cooking with the recipes you'll find in the following pages. They were created to fit the busy lifestyle virtually all of us lead today, and many can be prepared and on the table in around 30 minutes or less. (Dishes for entertaining or special celebrations are also included for occasions when you have more time to spend in the kitchen.) We've used everyday ingredients and simple preparations even first-time cooks can easily master. Best of all, every recipe follows the EATINGWELL philosophy of including a wide variety of healthy foods made with wholesome, minimally processed ingredients.

> **"No meal is so good as when you have your feet under your own table."**
>
> SCOTT NEARING

To keep you feeling satisfied, our recipes emphasize ample lean protein and low-fat dairy products (or their substitutes). Vegetables are found in abundance, and we encourage you to use fresh choices in season, when they're at the height of their flavor.

All our recipes meet the primary EATINGWELL criterion: they taste great and can be served to anyone without apology (and with high expectations of success). Enjoy every bite!

RECIPES

RECIPE GUIDELINES & NUTRIENT ANALYSES

DEFINING "ACTIVE MINUTES" AND "TOTAL":

Testers in the EATINGWELL Test Kitchen keep track of the time needed for each recipe. **Active Minutes** includes prep time (the time it takes to chop, dice, puree, mix, combine, etc. before cooking begins), but it also includes the time spent tending something on the stovetop, in the oven or on the grill—and getting it to the table. If you can't walk away from it, we consider it active minutes. **Total** includes both active and inactive minutes and indicates the entire amount of time required for each recipe, start to finish. **To Make Ahead** gives storage instructions to help you plan. If special **Equipment** is needed, we tell you that at the top of the recipe too.

ANALYSIS NOTES:

Each recipe is analyzed for calories, total fat, saturated (SAT) and monounsaturated (MONO) fat, cholesterol, carbohydrate, protein, fiber, sodium and potassium. (Numbers less than 0.5 are rounded down to 0; 0.5 to 0.9 are rounded up to 1.) We use Food Processor SQL software (ESHA Research) for analyses.

When a recipe states a measure of salt "or to taste," we analyze the measured quantity. (Readers on sodium-restricted diets can reduce or eliminate the salt.) Recipes are tested with iodized table salt unless otherwise indicated. Kosher or sea salt is called for when the recipe will benefit from the unique texture or flavor. We assume that rinsing with water reduces the sodium in canned beans by 35%.

Butter is analyzed as unsalted. We do not include trimmings or marinade that is not absorbed. When alternative ingredients are listed, we analyze the first one suggested. Optional ingredients and garnishes are not analyzed. Portion sizes are consistent with healthy-eating guidelines.

NUTRITION ICONS:

Our nutritionists have highlighted recipes likely to be of interest to those following various dietary plans. Recipes that meet specific guidelines are marked with these icons:

Healthy)(Weight

An entree has reduced calories, fats and saturated fats, as follows:

CALORIES ≤ **350**, TOTAL FAT ≤ **20g**, SAT FAT ≤ **5g**

Lower ⬇ Carbs

Recipe has 22 grams or less of carbohydrate per serving.

High ⬆ Fiber

Recipe provides 5 grams or more of fiber per serving.

NUTRITION BONUSES:

Nutrition bonuses are indicated for recipes that provide 15% or more of the daily value (dv) of specific nutrients. The daily values are the average daily recommended nutrient intakes for most adults that you see listed on food labels. In addition to the nutrients listed on food labels (vitamins A and C, calcium, iron and fiber), we have included bonus information for other nutrients, such as folate, magnesium, potassium, selenium and zinc, when a recipe is particularly high in one of these. We have chosen to highlight these nutrients because of their importance to good health and the fact that many Americans may have inadequate intakes of them.

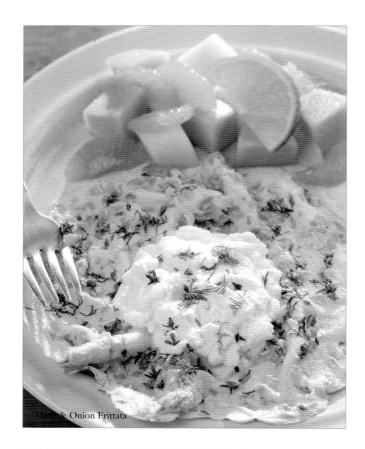

Herb & Onion Frittata

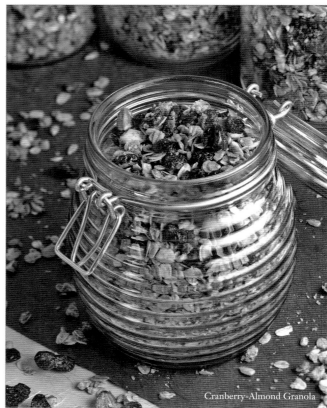

Cranberry-Almond Granola

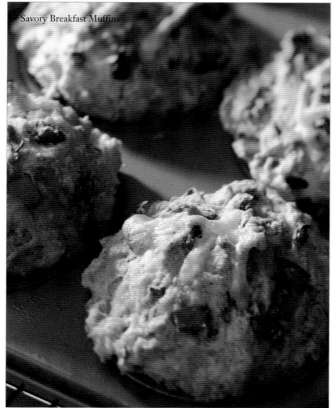

Savory Breakfast Muffins

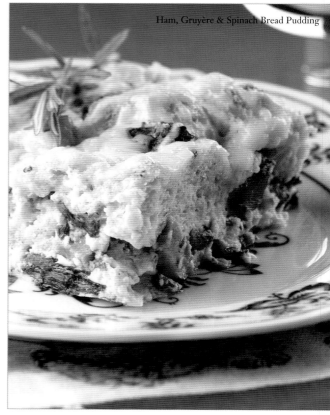

Ham, Gruyère & Spinach Bread Pudding

BREAKFAST

"I have to exercise in the morning
before my brain figures out what I'm doing.**"**
MARSHA DOBLE, COMEDIAN

198 CALORIES

9 g fat (3 g sat, 5 g mono)

20 mg cholesterol

7 g carbohydrate

24 g protein

3 g fiber

978 mg sodium

539 mg potassium

NUTRITION BONUS:
Vitamin A (25% daily value)
Folate (22% dv)
Selenium (21% dv)
Iron (20% dv)
Calcium, Potassium &
Vitamin C (15% dv)

Healthy)(Weight

Lower ⬇ Carbs

ACTIVE TIME: **10 MINUTES**

TOTAL: **10 MINUTES**

ASPARAGUS & CANADIAN BACON OMELET

An omelet is a satisfying meal to start the day, and will give you staying power until your midmorning snack. Although cooking a low-fat omelet may seem complicated at first glance, it will quickly become second nature.

- 10 stalks asparagus, trimmed and chopped
- ¼ cup plus 1 tablespoon water, divided
- 2 slices Canadian bacon, diced (1 ounce)
- 1 teaspoon extra-virgin olive oil
- ½ cup liquid egg substitute, such as Egg Beaters
- ¼ cup shredded reduced-fat Cheddar cheese
- ⅛ teaspoon salt
- ⅛ teaspoon freshly ground pepper

1. Bring asparagus and ¼ cup water to a boil in a small nonstick skillet over medium-high heat. Cover and cook until the asparagus is slightly softened, about 2 minutes. Uncover and continue cooking until the water has evaporated, 1 to 2 minutes.

2. Add Canadian bacon and oil to the pan and stir to coat. Pour in egg substitute, reduce heat to medium-low and continue cooking, stirring constantly with a heatproof rubber spatula, until the egg is starting to set, about 20 seconds. Continue cooking, lifting the edges so the uncooked egg will flow underneath, until mostly set, about 30 seconds more.

3. Sprinkle cheese, salt and pepper over the omelet. Lift up an edge of the omelet and drizzle the remaining 1 tablespoon water under it. Cover, reduce heat to low and cook until the egg is completely set and the cheese is melted, about 2 minutes. Fold over using the spatula and serve.

MAKES **1** SERVING.

HERB & ONION FRITTATA

This Italian-style omelet is delicious with just about any herb combination; try parsley, dill, chervil or marjoram.

1 cup diced onion
¼ cup plus 1 tablespoon water, divided
1 teaspoon extra-virgin olive oil
½ cup liquid egg substitute, such as Egg Beaters
2 teaspoons chopped fresh herbs *or* ½ teaspoon dried
⅛ teaspoon salt
⅛ teaspoon freshly ground pepper
2 tablespoons farmer's cheese *or* reduced-fat ricotta

1. Bring onion and ¼ cup water to a boil in a small nonstick skillet over medium-high heat. Cover and cook until the onion is slightly softened, about 2 minutes. Uncover and continue cooking until the water has evaporated, 1 to 2 minutes. Drizzle in oil and stir until coated. Continue cooking, stirring often, until the onion is beginning to brown, 1 to 2 minutes more.
2. Pour in egg substitute, reduce heat to medium-low and continue cooking, stirring constantly with a heatproof rubber spatula, until the egg is starting to set, about 20 seconds. Continue cooking, lifting the edges so the uncooked egg will flow underneath, until mostly set, about 30 seconds more.
3. Reduce heat to low. Sprinkle herbs, salt and pepper over the frittata. Spoon cheese on top. Lift up an edge of the frittata and drizzle the remaining 1 tablespoon water under it. Cover and cook until the egg is completely set and the cheese is hot, about 2 minutes. Slide the frittata out of the pan using the spatula and serve.

MAKES 1 SERVING.

PER SERVING:

192 CALORIES

7 g fat (2 g sat, 4 g mono)
10 mg cholesterol
17 g carbohydrate
15 g protein
3 g fiber
527 mg sodium
339 mg potassium

NUTRITION BONUS:
Vitamin C (20% daily value)

Healthy ⧓ Weight

Lower ⬇ Carbs

ACTIVE TIME: **10 MINUTES**

TOTAL: **10 MINUTES**

PER SERVING:

152 CALORIES

7 g fat (2 g sat, 4 g mono)

6 mg cholesterol

8 g carbohydrate

17 g protein

3 g fiber

619 mg sodium

362 mg potassium

NUTRITION BONUS:
Vitamin A (35% daily value)
Vitamin C (30% dv)
Calcium (15% dv)

Healthy)(Weight

Lower ↓ Carbs

ACTIVE TIME: **20 MINUTES**

TOTAL: **20 MINUTES**

SPINACH & TOMATO OMELET

This colorful, flavorful omelet packs two servings of vegetables. Now that's starting your day off right!

1	teaspoon extra-virgin olive oil
5	cherry tomatoes, halved
1	scallion, sliced
1	cup baby spinach, washed, with water still clinging to leaves
½	cup liquid egg substitute, such as Egg Beaters
¼	cup shredded reduced-fat Cheddar cheese
⅛	teaspoon salt
⅛	teaspoon freshly ground pepper
1	tablespoon water

1. Spray a small nonstick skillet with cooking spray. Add oil and heat over medium-high heat. Add tomatoes and scallion and cook, stirring once or twice, until softened, 1 to 2 minutes. Place spinach on top, cover and let wilt, about 30 seconds. Stir to combine.

2. Pour in egg substitute, reduce heat to medium-low and continue cooking, stirring constantly with a heatproof rubber spatula, until the egg is starting to set, about 20 seconds. Continue cooking, lifting the edges so the uncooked egg will flow underneath, until mostly set, about 30 seconds more.

3. Sprinkle cheese, salt and pepper over the omelet. Lift up an edge of the omelet and drizzle the remaining 1 tablespoon water under it. Cover, reduce heat to low and cook until the egg is completely set and the cheese is melted, about 2 minutes. Fold over using the spatula and serve.

MAKES **1** SERVING.

HAM, GRUYÈRE & SPINACH BREAD PUDDING

High-quality ham is worth the cost. It infuses the pudding with a smoky flavor that compliments the spinach, peppers, rosemary and Gruyère.

4	large egg whites
4	large eggs
1	cup skim milk
2	tablespoons Dijon mustard
1	teaspoon minced fresh rosemary
1/4	teaspoon freshly ground pepper
4	cups whole-grain bread, crusts removed if desired, cut into 1-inch cubes (about 1/2 pound, 4-6 slices)
5	cups chopped spinach, wilted (*see Tip*)
1	cup diced ham steak (5 ounces)
1/2	cup chopped jarred roasted red peppers
3/4	cup shredded Gruyère cheese

1. Preheat oven to 375°F. Coat an 11-by-7-inch glass baking dish or a 2-quart casserole with cooking spray.

2. Whisk egg whites, eggs and milk in a medium bowl. Add mustard, rosemary and pepper; whisk to combine.

3. Toss bread, spinach, ham and peppers in a large bowl. Add the egg mixture and toss well to coat. Transfer to the prepared baking dish and push down to compact. Cover with foil.

4. Bake until the custard has set, 40 to 45 minutes. Uncover, sprinkle with cheese and continue baking until the pudding is puffed and golden on top, 15 to 20 minutes more. Transfer to a wire rack and cool for 15 to 20 minutes before serving.

MAKES **6** SERVINGS.

PER SERVING:

276 CALORIES

10 g fat (4 g sat, 3 g mono)
169 mg cholesterol
25 g carbohydrate
21 g protein
3 g fiber
746 mg sodium
422 mg potassium

NUTRITION BONUS:
Vitamin A (70% daily value)
Folate (37% dv)
Calcium (30% dv)
Vitamin C (20% dv)

Healthy ⨉ Weight

ACTIVE TIME: **30 MINUTES**

TOTAL: 1 3/4 **HOURS**

TO MAKE AHEAD: **Prepare the pudding through Step 3; refrigerate overnight. Let stand at room temperature while the oven preheats. Bake as directed in Step 4.**

TO WILT GREENS:

- Rinse greens thoroughly. Transfer them to a large microwave-safe bowl. Cover with plastic wrap and punch several holes in it. Microwave on High until wilted, 2 to 3 minutes. Squeeze out any excess moisture from the greens before adding them to the recipe.

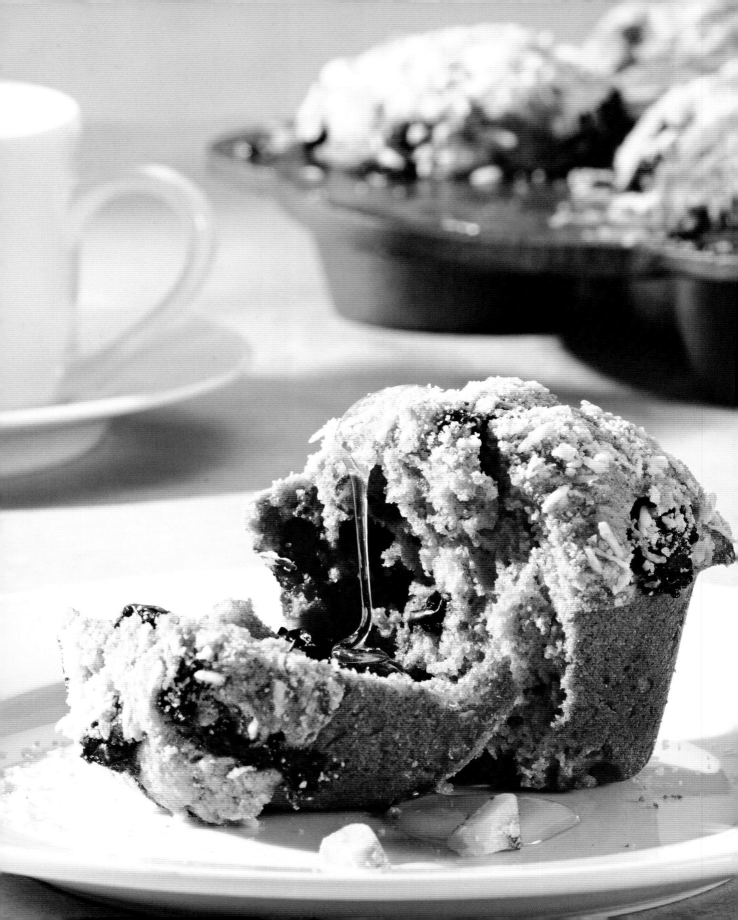

BLUEBERRY-COCONUT-MACADAMIA MUFFINS

The one-two punch of coconut and macadamia nuts in this luxurious muffin will make you think you're having your morning coffee in Hawaii. Drizzle with honey for an added touch of sweetness.

- ¼ cup unsweetened coconut
- 2 tablespoons plus ¾ cup all-purpose flour, divided
- 2 tablespoons plus ½ cup brown sugar, divided
- 5 tablespoons chopped macadamia nuts, divided
- 2 tablespoons canola oil, divided
- 1 cup whole-wheat pastry flour (*see page 245*) *or* whole-wheat flour
- 1 teaspoon baking powder
- ¼ teaspoon baking soda
- ⅛ teaspoon salt
- ½ teaspoon ground cinnamon
- 1 large egg
- 1 large egg white
- ¾ cup nonfat buttermilk (*see Tip, page 245*)
- 2 tablespoons butter, melted
- ½ teaspoon coconut *or* vanilla extract
- 1 ½ cups fresh *or* frozen (*not* thawed) blueberries

1. Preheat oven to 400°F. Coat a 12-cup muffin pan with cooking spray.

2. Combine coconut, 2 tablespoons all-purpose flour, 2 tablespoons brown sugar and 2 tablespoons macadamia nuts in a small bowl. Drizzle with 1 tablespoon oil; stir to combine. Set aside.

3. Whisk the remaining ¾ cup all-purpose flour, whole-wheat flour, baking powder, baking soda, salt and cinnamon in a medium bowl. Whisk the remaining ½ cup brown sugar, the remaining 1 tablespoon oil, egg, egg white, buttermilk, butter and coconut (or vanilla) extract in a medium bowl until well combined. Make a well in the center of the dry ingredients and pour in the wet ingredients; stir until just combined. Add blueberries and the remaining 3 tablespoons nuts; stir just to combine. Divide the batter among the prepared muffin cups. Sprinkle with the reserved coconut topping and gently press into the batter.

4. Bake the muffins until golden brown and a wooden skewer inserted in the center comes out clean, about 20 minutes. Let cool in the pan for 10 minutes, then remove from the pan and let cool on a wire rack at least 5 minutes more before serving.

MAKES **1** DOZEN MUFFINS.

ACTIVE TIME: **20 MINUTES**

TOTAL: **45 MINUTES**

INGREDIENT NOTE:

■ You can use buttermilk powder in place of fresh buttermilk. Or make "sour milk": mix 1 tablespoon lemon juice or vinegar to 1 cup milk.

SAVORY BREAKFAST MUFFINS

If you like to start your day with bold flavors, here's your ideal grab-and-go breakfast: The smoky bacon, Cheddar and peppery heat will really stoke your furnace, and the ample protein content will help you feel satisfied all morning. Serve them warm.

2 cups whole-wheat flour
1 cup all-purpose flour
1 tablespoon baking powder
½ teaspoon baking soda
½ teaspoon freshly ground pepper
¼ teaspoon salt
2 large eggs
1⅓ cups buttermilk *or* equivalent buttermilk powder (*see Note*)
3 tablespoons extra-virgin olive oil
2 tablespoons butter, melted
1 cup thinly sliced scallions (about 1 bunch)
¾ cup diced Canadian bacon (3 ounces)
½ cup grated Cheddar cheese
½ cup finely diced red bell pepper

1. Preheat oven to 400°F. Coat 12 standard 2½-inch muffin cups with cooking spray.
2. Combine whole-wheat flour, all-purpose flour, baking powder, baking soda, pepper and salt in a large bowl.
3. Whisk eggs, buttermilk, oil and butter in a medium bowl. Fold in scallions, bacon, cheese and bell pepper. Make a well in the center of the dry ingredients. Add the wet ingredients and mix with a rubber spatula until just moistened. Scoop the batter into the prepared pan (the cups will be very full).
4. Bake the muffins until the tops are golden brown, 20 to 22 minutes. Let cool in the pan for 5 minutes. Loosen the edges and turn the muffins out onto a wire rack to cool slightly before serving.

MAKES **1** DOZEN MUFFINS.

CRANBERRY-ALMOND GRANOLA

If you've never made your own granola, you'll be amazed at the difference in freshness and flavor—and at how easy it is. Use this recipe as a starting point for your own creativity: substitute dried blueberries or chopped dried apricots for the cranberries, or walnuts or hazelnuts for the almonds.

2/3	cup frozen unsweetened apple juice concentrate, thawed
1/2	cup maple syrup
1/3	cup almond oil *or* canola oil
1/4	cup packed dark brown sugar
1	tablespoon ground cinnamon
1/2	teaspoon salt, or to taste
5	cups rolled oats (*not* quick-cooking)
1	cup toasted wheat germ
1	cup whole almonds, coarsely chopped (4 1/2 ounces)
1/2	cup sunflower seeds (2 ounces)
1	cup dried cranberries, divided

1. Position racks in the top and bottom thirds of the oven; preheat to 325°F. Coat 2 large baking sheets with sides with cooking spray.

2. Whisk apple juice concentrate, maple syrup, oil and brown sugar in a medium saucepan. Bring to a simmer over medium-high heat, stirring occasionally. Remove from heat; stir in cinnamon and salt.

3. Mix oats, wheat germ, almonds and sunflower seeds in a large bowl. Stir in the juice mixture; toss to coat. Spread the granola evenly on the prepared baking sheets.

4. Bake the granola for 15 minutes, stirring once or twice. Reverse sheets top to bottom and back to front. Continue baking until lightly browned and aromatic, stirring frequently, about 15 minutes more. Transfer the baking sheets to wire racks; stir 1/2 cup dried cranberries into the granola on each sheet. Let cool completely.

MAKES 9 1/2 CUPS (19 SERVINGS, 1/2 CUP EACH).

PER SERVING:

262 CALORIES

11 g fat (1 g sat, 6 g mono)

0 mg cholesterol

37 g carbohydrate

7 g protein

5 g fiber

67 mg sodium

229 mg potassium

NUTRITION BONUS:
Magnesium & Fiber (20% daily value)

Healthy)(Weight

High ⬆ Fiber

ACTIVE TIME: **10 MINUTES**

TOTAL: **2 HOURS (with cooling)**

EASY BREAKFASTS

Banana-Cocoa Soy Smoothie

Slice a banana and freeze until firm. Blend ½ cup silken tofu, ½ cup soymilk, 2 tablespoons unsweetened cocoa powder and 1 tablespoon honey in a blender until smooth. With the motor running, add the banana slices through the hole in the lid and continue to puree until smooth.
MAKES 1 SERVING.
PER SERVING: 340 calories; 8 g fat (1 g sat, 1 g mono); 0 mg cholesterol; 60 g carbohydrate; 17 g protein; 10 g fiber; 121 mg sodium; 749 mg potassium. NUTRITION BONUS: Magnesium (29% daily value), Potassium (21% dv), Iron (20% dv), Vitamin A & Vitamin C (15% dv).

Breakfast Parfait

Top ¾ cup low-fat cottage cheese or ¾ cup low-fat plain yogurt with 1 cup pineapple chunks, papaya chunks or cling peaches. Sprinkle with 2 teaspoons toasted wheat germ.
MAKES 1 SERVING.
PER SERVING (with cottage cheese, pineapple): 248 calories; 2 g fat (1 g sat, 1 g mono); 7 mg cholesterol; 35 g carbohydrate; 23 g protein; 3 g fiber; 24 mg sodium; 414 mg potassium. NUTRITION BONUS: Vitamin C (30% daily value), Selenium (20% dv), Calcium (15% dv).

PER SERVING (with yogurt, papaya): 185 calories; 3 g fat (2 g sat, 0 g mono); 15 mg cholesterol; 28 g carbohydrate; 10 g protein; 3 g fiber; 132 mg sodium; 404 mg potassium. NUTRITION BONUS: Vitamin C (150% daily value), Vitamin A (40% dv), Calcium (35% dv), Folate (17% dv).

Breakfast Pigs in a Blanket

Heat 2 frozen pancakes (preferably whole-grain) in the microwave to soften for about 30 seconds. Spread 1 teaspoon raspberry jam down the center of each. Place one ½-ounce slice of ham on each. Microwave to heat through, about 1 minute. Roll up.
MAKES 1 SERVING.

PER SERVING: 203 calories; 5 g fat (1 g sat, 1 g mono); 29 mg cholesterol; 31 g carbohydrate; 10 g protein; 1 g fiber; 275 mg sodium; 103 mg potassium.

Cheddar-Apple Melt

Toast 1 whole-wheat English muffin. Top with 2 teaspoons jam or chutney, thin slices of apple and 2 slices reduced-fat Cheddar cheese. Toast in a toaster oven or under the broiler until the cheese is melted.
MAKES 1 SERVING.
PER SERVING: 253 calories; 5 g fat (3 g sat, 2 g mono); 12 mg cholesterol; 33 g carbohydrate; 20 g protein; 5 g fiber; 769 mg sodium; 215 mg potassium. NUTRITION BONUS: Selenium (50% daily value), Calcium (40% dv), Magnesium (15%).

EatingWell Diet Breakfast Smoothie

Puree 1 cup nonfat vanilla yogurt with ¼ cup fruit juice in a blender until smooth. With the motor running, add 1½ cups (6½ ounces) frozen fruit, such as blueberries, raspberries, pineapple or peaches, through the hole in the lid and continue to puree until smooth.
MAKES 1 SERVING.
PER SERVING: 355 calories; 0 g fat (0 g sat, 0 g mono); 4 mg cholesterol; 74 g carbohydrate; 14 g protein; 6 g fiber; 170 mg sodium; 559 mg potassium. NUTRITION BONUS: Vitamin C (80% daily value), Calcium (46% dv), Potassium (16% dv).

Peanut Butter-Cinnamon English Muffin

Toast 1 whole-wheat English muffin. Meanwhile combine 1 teaspoon sugar with ¼ teaspoon cinnamon. Spread 1 tablespoon peanut butter on the toasted muffin. Sprinkle with the cinnamon sugar.
MAKES 1 SERVING.
PER SERVING: 247 calories; 9 g fat (2 g sat, 4 g mono); 0 mg cholesterol; 35 g carbohydrate; 10 g protein; 6 g fiber; 496 mg sodium; 246 mg potassium. NUTRITION BONUS: Selenium (40% daily value), Magnesium (18% dv), Calcium (20% dv).

Quick Breakfast Taco

Top 2 corn tortillas with 1 tablespoon salsa and 2 tablespoons shredded reduced-fat Cheddar cheese. Heat in the microwave until the cheese is melted, about 30 seconds. Meanwhile coat a small nonstick skillet with cooking spray. Heat over medium heat, add ½ cup liquid egg substitute, such as Egg Beaters, and cook, stirring, until the eggs are cooked through, about 90 seconds. Divide the scrambled egg between the tacos.

MAKES 1 SERVING.

PER SERVING: 123 calories; 2 g fat (1 g sat, 0 g mono); 3 mg cholesterol; 13 g carbohydrate; 13 g protein; 0 g fiber; 295 mg sodium; 137 mg potassium.

Raisin Bread & Farmer's Cheese

Toast 2 slices whole-wheat raisin bread. Spread with 4 tablespoons farmer's cheese *or* part-skim ricotta cheese. Drizzle with 1 teaspoon honey.

MAKES 1 SERVING.

PER SERVING (with farmer's cheese): 243 calories; 7 g fat (4 g sat, 1 g mono); 20 mg cholesterol; 27 g carbohydrate; 14 g protein; 2 g fiber; 444 mg sodium; 118 mg potassium. NUTRITION BONUS: Folate (18% daily value). PER SERVING (with ricotta): 228 calories; 7 g fat (4 g sat, 3 g mono); 19 mg cholesterol; 31 g carbohydrate; 11 g protein; 2 g fiber; 281 mg sodium; 196 mg potassium. NUTRITION BONUS: Selenium (30% daily value), Calcium & Folate (20% dv).

Tomato & Ham Breakfast Melt

Toast 2 slices of thin multigrain bread, such as Pepperidge Farm "thin." Top with 4 thin slices tomato, 4 thin slices ham and 2 slices reduced-fat Cheddar cheese. Toast in a toaster oven or under the broiler until the cheese is melted.

MAKES 1 SERVING.

PER SERVING: 299 calories; 10 g fat (4 g sat, 3 g mono); 48 mg cholesterol; 25 g carbohydrate; 31 g protein; 7 g fiber; 1,129 mg sodium; 522 mg potassium. NUTRITION BONUS: Calcium (30% daily value), Selenium (25% dv), Zinc (24% dv), Vitamin C (20% dv), Magnesium (17% dv), Iron & Vitamin A (15% dv).

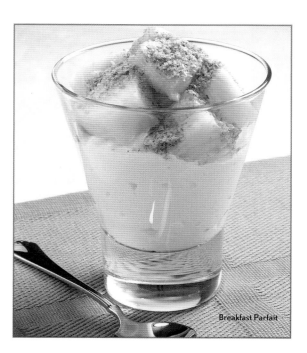

Breakfast Parfait

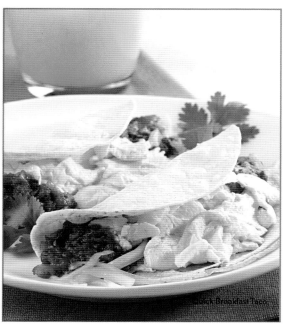

Quick Breakfast Taco

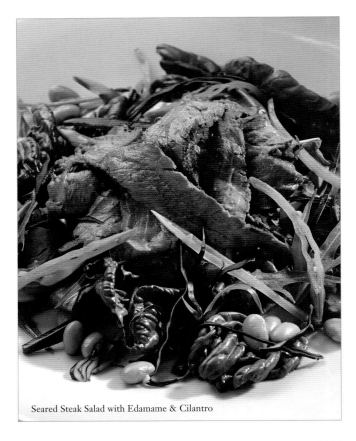

Seared Steak Salad with Edamame & Cilantro

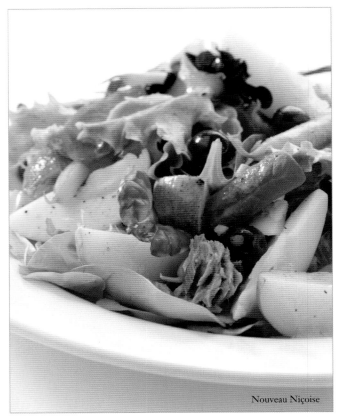

Nouveau Niçoise

Shrimp Caesar

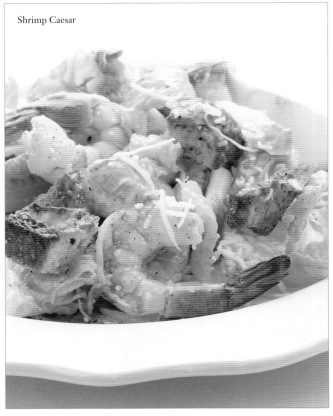

EatingWell Power Salad

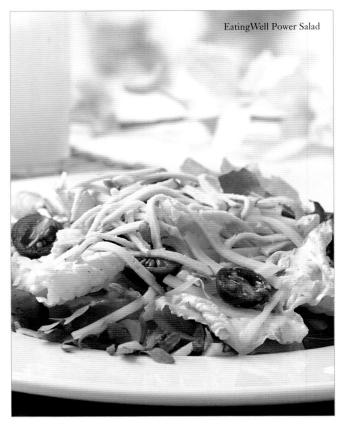

SALADS

> **"**I don't altogether agree that a plain green salad ever becomes a bore—not, that is, if it's made with fresh, well-drained crisp green stuff and a properly seasoned dressing of good-quality olive oil and a sound wine vinegar.**"**
>
> ELIZABETH DAVID, COOKBOOK AUTHOR

PER SERVING:

300 CALORIES

13 g fat (3 g sat, 6 g mono)

216 mg cholesterol

26 g carbohydrate

22 g protein

8 g fiber

823 mg sodium

592 mg potassium

NUTRITION BONUS:
Vitamin A (240% daily value)
Folate (35% dv)
Vitamin C (30% dv)
Calcium (15% dv)

Healthy)(Weight

High ⬆ Fiber

ACTIVE TIME: **20 MINUTES**

TOTAL: **30 MINUTES**

LOADED SPINACH SALAD

Like many spinach salads, this one features lots of chopped-up hard-boiled egg. But since most of the calories in an egg are in the yolk, we use just two whole eggs, plus the whites from six additional eggs. The result is a rich, eggy, satisfying spinach salad that keeps the calories in check.

8	eggs
6	cups baby spinach
4	tablespoons Creamy Blue Cheese Dressing (*page 127*), divided
1	8-ounce can beets, rinsed and sliced
1	cup shredded carrots
2	tablespoons chopped pecans, toasted (*see Tip, page 245*)

Place eggs in a single layer in a saucepan; cover with water. Bring to a simmer over medium-high heat. Reduce heat to low, cover and cook at the lowest simmer for 10 minutes. Pour off the hot water and run cold water over the eggs until they are completely cooled. Peel the eggs, discard 6 of the yolks, chop the remaining yolks and whites. Toss spinach and 2 tablespoons dressing in a large bowl. Divide between 2 plates. Top with chopped eggs, beets, carrots and pecans. Drizzle with the remaining 2 tablespoons dressing.

MAKES **2** SERVINGS, ABOUT **4** CUPS EACH.

THE EATINGWELL
COBB SALAD

Originally developed at a Hollywood restaurant, this classic salad has endured endless interpretation. Our version is fairly true to the original, although we've left the blue cheese optional. Make it a meal: Warm up a crusty baguette and pour a crisp, cold glass of sparkling wine to accompany this salad.

- 3 tablespoons white-wine vinegar
- 2 tablespoons finely minced shallot
- 1 tablespoon Dijon mustard
- 1/4 teaspoon salt
- 1 teaspoon freshly ground pepper
- 3 tablespoons extra-virgin olive oil
- 10 cups mixed salad greens
- 1/2 pound shredded cooked chicken breast (1 large breast half) (*see Tip*)
- 2 eggs, hard-boiled, peeled and chopped (*see Tip, page 245*)
- 2 strips bacon, cooked and crumbled
- 2 medium tomatoes, diced
- 1 large cucumber, seeded and sliced
- 1 avocado, diced
- 1/2 cup crumbled blue cheese (optional)

1. Whisk vinegar, shallot, mustard, salt and pepper in a small bowl to combine. Whisk in oil until combined. Place salad greens in a large bowl. Add half of the dressing and toss to coat.

2. Divide salad greens among 4 plates. Arrange equal portions of chicken, egg, bacon, tomatoes, cucumber, avocado and blue cheese (if using) on top of the lettuce. Drizzle the salads with the remaining dressing.

MAKES 4 SERVINGS, ABOUT 4 CUPS EACH.

PER SERVING:

314 CALORIES

23 g fat (4 g sat, 15 g mono)
127 mg cholesterol
15 g carbohydrate
16 g protein
8 g fiber
364 mg sodium
1,077 mg potassium

NUTRITION BONUS:
Vitamin A (90% daily value)
Vitamin C (60% dv)
Potassium (31% dv)
Iron (20% dv)

Lower ⬇ Carbs

High ⬆ Fiber

ACTIVE TIME: **40 MINUTES**

TOTAL: **40 MINUTES**

TIP:

- To poach chicken breasts, place boneless, skinless breasts in a medium skillet or saucepan and add enough water to cover; bring to a boil. Cover, reduce heat to low and simmer gently until the chicken is cooked through and no longer pink in the middle, 10 to 12 minutes.

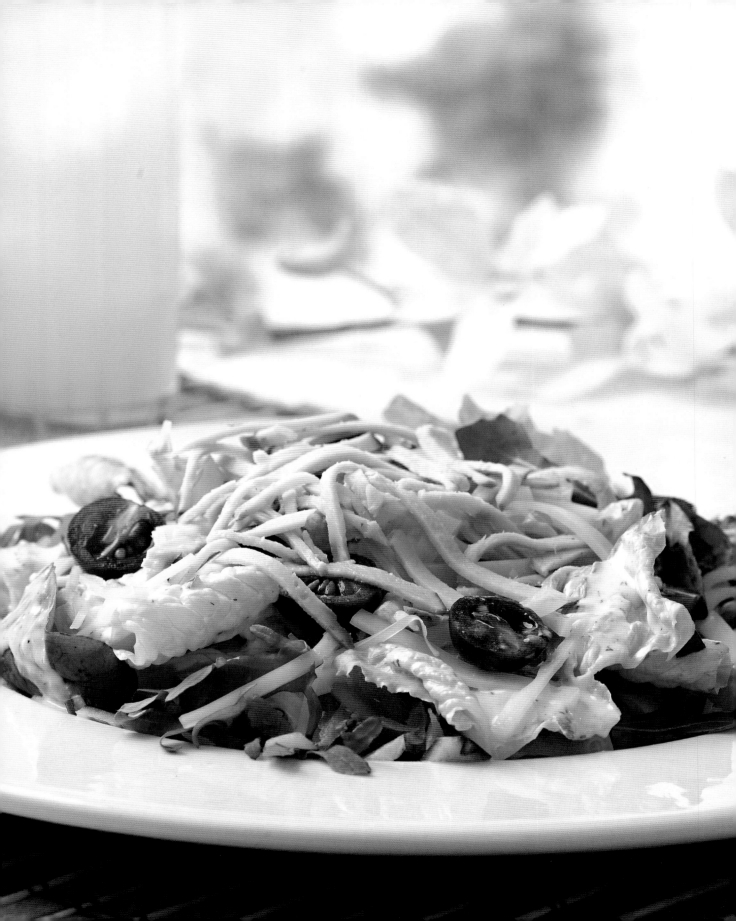

EATINGWELL POWER SALAD

Here's our take on a traditional chef's salad, which is anything but light fare when it's heaped with meats and cheeses. Our version keeps the satisfaction factor with lean turkey breast and reduced-fat Swiss cheese—and adds plenty of colorful vegetables to the mix.

6	cups mixed greens
1	cup shredded carrots
2	tablespoons chopped red onion
¼	cup dressing, such as Creamy Dill Ranch Dressing (*page 126*)
10	cherry tomatoes
4	slices roast turkey breast, cut up (3 ounces)
2	slices reduced-fat Swiss cheese, cut up (2 ounces)

Toss greens, carrots, onion and dressing in a large bowl until coated. Divide between 2 plates. Arrange tomatoes, turkey and cheese on top of the salad.

MAKES 2 SERVINGS, ABOUT 4 CUPS EACH.

PER SERVING:

180 CALORIES

4 g fat (1 g sat, 0 g mono)

27 mg cholesterol

19 g carbohydrate

21 g protein

6 g fiber

757 mg sodium

956 mg potassium

NUTRITION BONUS:
Vitamin A (290% daily value)
Vitamin C (70% dv)
Folate (55% dv)
Calcium (40% dv)

Healthy)(Weight

Lower ⬇ Carbs

High ⬆ Fiber

ACTIVE TIME: **10 MINUTES**

TOTAL: **10 MINUTES**

242 CALORIES

5 g fat (2 g sat, 2 g mono)

8 mg cholesterol

38 g carbohydrate

13 g protein

15 g fiber

621 mg sodium

1,059 mg potassium

NUTRITION BONUS:
Vitamin A (200% daily value)
Vitamin C (160% dv)
Folate (84% dv)
Calcium (20% dv)

Healthy ⋈ Weight

High ⬆ Fiber

ACTIVE TIME: **15 MINUTES**

TOTAL: **15 MINUTES**

TIP:

- Store leftover canned beans in the refrigerator for up to 3 days. Toss them into soup for extra protein; mash with garlic powder and chopped fresh herbs for a quick dip.

ROMAINE SALAD WITH ORANGE, FETA & BEANS

Adding canned beans is a quick, convenient way to make a salad into a meal—they boost the protein to make the salad more satisfying. We call for kidney beans, but other canned beans like cannellinis or black beans would also work nicely.

6	cups chopped romaine lettuce
1	cup sliced radishes
1	cup canned kidney beans, rinsed (*see Tip*)
1	orange, segmented
1	scallion, sliced
¼	cup crumbled reduced-fat feta cheese
¼	cup Orange-Oregano Dressing (*page 127*)

Combine lettuce, radishes, beans, orange, scallion, feta and dressing in a large bowl. Toss to coat.

MAKES **2** SERVINGS, ABOUT **4** CUPS EACH.

NOUVEAU NIÇOISE

This quick, easy remake of the Provençal standard turns a couple of cans of tuna into a main-course salad that's elegant enough for company.

8	cups water
8	ounces green beans, trimmed and halved
8	small red potatoes
2	eggs
¼	cup minced shallots
¼	cup red-wine vinegar
2	tablespoons Dijon mustard
¼	teaspoon salt
¼	teaspoon freshly ground pepper
3	tablespoons extra-virgin olive oil
6	cups mixed salad greens
2	6-ounce cans chunk light tuna, drained
12	Niçoise *or* Kalamata olives

1. Bring water to a boil in a 3- to 4-quart saucepan. Add green beans and cook until just tender and bright green, 1 to 2 minutes. Using a slotted spoon, transfer the beans to a colander, rinse under cold water and set aside in a large bowl. Carefully place potatoes and eggs into the boiling water. Cook the eggs until hard, 10 minutes. Using a slotted spoon, transfer the eggs to the colander, rinse under cold water until cool and set aside. Continue cooking the potatoes until fork-tender, 3 minutes more. Drain the potatoes; rinse under cold water until cool enough to handle.

2. Meanwhile, combine shallots, vinegar, mustard, salt and pepper in a small bowl. Slowly whisk in oil.

3. Cut the potatoes into quarters or eighths, depending on their size. Add to the bowl with the beans. Add greens, tuna and the dressing. Toss well. Peel the eggs and cut into wedges. Divide the salad among 4 plates. Top with egg wedges and olives. Serve immediately.

MAKES 4 SERVINGS, GENEROUS 2 CUPS EACH.

PER SERVING:

436 CALORIES

16 g fat (3 g sat, 11 g mono)

159 mg cholesterol

38 g carbohydrate

33 g protein

6 g fiber

547 mg sodium

1,139 mg potassium

NUTRITION BONUS:
Vitamin C (90% daily value)
Potassium (33% dv)
Vitamin A (30% dv)
Folate (26% dv)
Iron (15% dv)

High ⬆ Fiber

ACTIVE TIME: **30 MINUTES**

TOTAL: **40 MINUTES**

TO MAKE AHEAD: **Cook green beans, potatoes and eggs; dry, cover and refrigerate for up to 1 day.**

328 CALORIES

9 g fat (2 g sat, 3 g mono)

68 mg cholesterol

19 g carbohydrate

42 g protein

7 g fiber

678 mg sodium

949 mg potassium

NUTRITION BONUS:
Vitamin C (320% daily value)
Vitamin A (120% dv)
Zinc (46% dv)
Folate (43% dv)
Iron (35% dv)

Healthy ⚖ Weight

Lower ⬇ Carbs

High ⬆ Fiber

ACTIVE TIME: **25 MINUTES**

TOTAL: **30 MINUTES**

TO MAKE AHEAD: **Prepare through Step 1; refrigerate for up to 1 day.**

SEARED STEAK SALAD WITH EDAMAME & CILANTRO

Look for prewashed packages of Asian-style salad mixes at your supermarket—their peppery, exotic character is great with this full-flavored steak and dressing. Look for fiber- and protein-rich edamame (green soybeans) in the frozen vegetables section of your supermarket.

8	ounces top round steak, ¾ inch thick, trimmed of fat
½	teaspoon kosher salt
½	teaspoon freshly ground pepper
4	cups mixed Asian greens *or* mesclun greens
1	cup sliced snow peas
1	cup sliced red bell pepper
½	cup shredded red cabbage
½	cup chopped cilantro leaves
⅓	cup thawed shelled edamame
¼	cup Sesame Tamari Vinaigrette (*page 126*)

1. Sprinkle steak with salt and pepper. Coat a small nonstick skillet with cooking spray; place over medium heat. Add the steak and cook about 4 minutes per side for medium-rare. Let rest for (at least 5) minutes before slicing.

2. Combine greens, snow peas, bell pepper, cabbage, cilantro, edamame and vinaigrette in a large bowl. Toss to coat. Divide between 2 plates. Top with the steak.

MAKES **2** SERVINGS, **3** CUPS EACH.

CHICKEN VARIATION

Substitute 8 ounces chicken tenders for the steak. Cook through, 3 to 4 minutes per side.

PER SERVING: 233 CALORIES; 4 g fat (0 g sat, 1 g mono); 67 mg cholesterol; 19 g carbohydrate; 32 g protein; 7 g fiber; 678 mg sodium; 651 mg potassium.

SHRIMP VARIATION

Substitute 8 ounces cooked, peeled shrimp for the steak (omit Step 1).

PER SERVING: 241 CALORIES; 5 g fat (1 g sat, 1 g mono); 221 mg cholesterol; 19 g carbohydrate; 30 g protein; 7 g fiber; 884 mg sodium; 857 mg potassium.

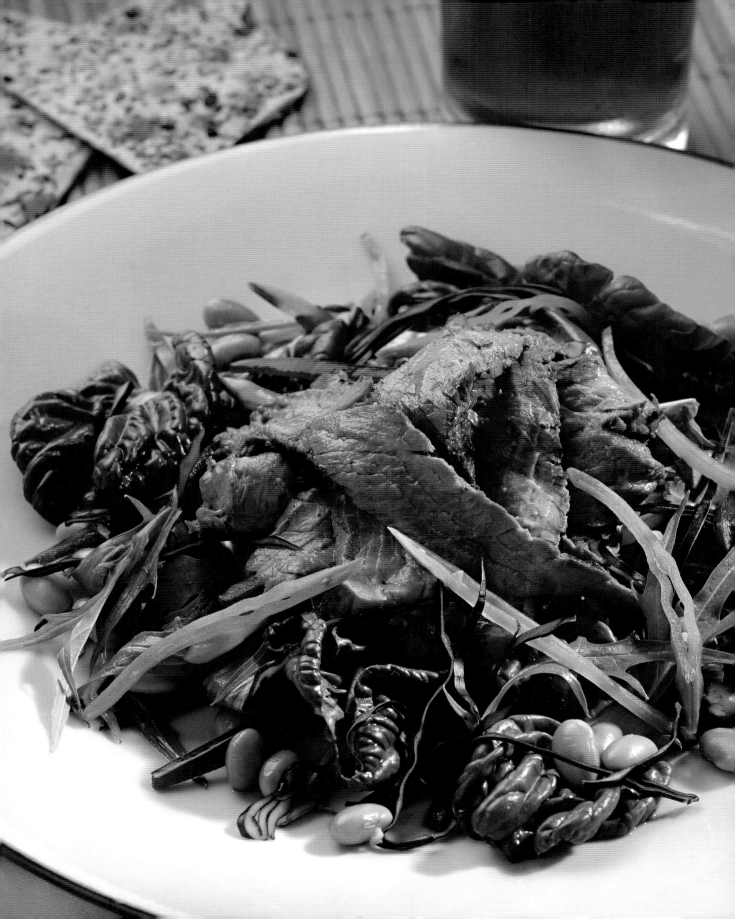

339 CALORIES

17 g fat (4 g sat, 8 g mono)

241 mg cholesterol

13 g carbohydrate

35 g protein

2 g fiber

749 mg sodium

368 mg potassium

NUTRITION BONUS:
Vitamin A (50% daily value)
Vitamin C (45% dv)
Iron (30% dv)
Calcium (20% dv)

Healthy ⅹ Weight

Lower ⬇ Carbs

ACTIVE TIME: **20 MINUTES**

TOTAL: **20 MINUTES**

TO MAKE AHEAD: **The
dressing (Step 1) will keep,
in a jar in the refrigerator, for
up to 3 days. Shake
vigorously just before tossing
with the salad.**

HOMEMADE CROUTONS:

▪ Toss 1 cup whole-grain
bread cubes with 1 table-
spoon extra-virgin olive oil,
a pinch each of salt, pepper
and garlic powder. Spread
out on a baking sheet and
toast at 350°F until crispy,
turning occasionally, 15 to
20 minutes.

SHRIMP CAESAR

*While most Caesars drown the greens in a heavy dressing, this lemony version lets
the taste of the shrimp shine through. Don't worry about the anchovies—they'll
mellow in the dressing, giving it a rich taste that can't be duplicated.*

3 tablespoons lemon juice, plus 4 lemon wedges for garnish
2 teaspoons Dijon mustard
3 anchovies, coarsely chopped, *or* 1 teaspoon anchovy paste,
 or to taste
1 small clove garlic, coarsely chopped
2 tablespoons extra-virgin olive oil
½ cup grated Asiago cheese, divided
½ teaspoon freshly ground pepper
8 cups chopped hearts of romaine (about 2 hearts)
1 pound peeled cooked shrimp (21-25 per pound; thawed if frozen)
1 cup croutons, preferably whole-grain (*see Tip*)

1. Place lemon juice, mustard, anchovies (or anchovy paste) and garlic in a
food processor; process until smooth. With the motor running, gradually
add oil; process until creamy. Add ¼ cup Asiago cheese and pepper; pulse
until combined.
2. Combine romaine, shrimp and croutons in a large bowl. Add the dressing and toss to coat. Divide among 4 plates, top with the remaining ¼ cup
Asiago cheese and garnish with a lemon wedge.

MAKES 4 SERVINGS, ABOUT 2 ½ CUPS EACH.

WARM SALAD OF GREENS, ITALIAN SAUSAGE & POTATOES

For a milder flavor, substitute escarole or Swiss chard for the mustard greens or kale (add them with the potatoes).

1	pound mustard greens *or* kale (about 12 cups packed), trimmed, washed and coarsely chopped
1	pound new potatoes, scrubbed and cut into ¾-inch chunks
½	pound hot *or* sweet Italian sausage, casing removed
2	teaspoons fennel seeds
2	tablespoons extra-virgin olive oil
2	tablespoons red-wine vinegar
1	small clove garlic, minced
¼	teaspoon salt, or to taste
	Freshly ground pepper to taste

1. Bring 2 cups lightly salted water to a boil in a large wide pan. Add mustard greens (or kale), cover and cook over medium heat for 5 minutes. Stir in potatoes; add about ½ cup water, if needed. Cover and cook until the potatoes and greens are tender, 5 to 10 minutes longer. Drain and place in a large bowl.

2. Meanwhile, cook sausage with fennel seeds in a small skillet over medium heat, turning from time to time, until cooked through, 10 to 12 minutes. (The seeds will adhere to the sausage.) Drain. Cut sausage into ½-inch-thick slices; add to the potato mixture.

3. Whisk oil, vinegar, garlic, salt and pepper in a small bowl. Pour over the sausage-potato mixture and toss to blend. Serve immediately.

MAKES 4 SERVINGS, 1¼ CUPS EACH.

PER SERVING:

262 CALORIES

15 g fat (4 g sat, 9 g mono)
16 mg cholesterol
23 g carbohydrate
10 g protein
4 g fiber
952 mg sodium
655 mg potassium

NUTRITION BONUS:
Vitamin A (110% daily value)
Vitamin C (60% dv)
Folate & Potassium (19% dv)

Healthy)(Weight

ACTIVE TIME: **25 MINUTES**

TOTAL: **50 MINUTES**

262 CALORIES

11 g fat (1 g sat, 5 g mono)

71 mg cholesterol

16 g carbohydrate

27 g protein

2 g fiber

706 mg sodium

349 mg potassium

NUTRITION BONUS:
Vitamin C (32% daily value)
Excellent source of omega-3s

Healthy)(Weight

Lower ⬇ Carbs

ACTIVE TIME: **25 MINUTES**

TOTAL: **25 MINUTES**

WARM SALMON SALAD WITH CRISPY POTATOES

We've stretched the definition of salad here, deliciously. In this updated homage to rösti (the famous Swiss potato pancake), this light salad starts with a bed of crispy potatoes and includes some delicious fish, flavorful greens and a perk-you-up dressing.

- 2 tablespoons extra-virgin olive oil, divided
- 2 small yellow-fleshed potatoes, such as Yukon Gold, scrubbed and cut into ⅛-inch slices
- ½ teaspoon salt, divided
- 1 medium shallot, thinly sliced
- 2 teaspoons rice vinegar
- ¼ cup buttermilk
- 2 7-ounce cans boneless, skinless salmon, drained
- 4 cups arugula

1. Heat 1 tablespoon oil in a large nonstick skillet over medium-high heat. Add potatoes and cook, turning once, until brown and crispy, 5 to 6 minutes per side. Transfer to a plate and season with ¼ teaspoon salt; cover with foil to keep warm.

2. Combine the remaining 1 tablespoon oil, ¼ teaspoon salt, shallot and vinegar in a small saucepan. Bring to a boil over medium heat. Remove from the heat and whisk in buttermilk. Place salmon in a medium bowl and toss with the warm dressing. Divide arugula among 4 plates and top with the potatoes and salmon.

MAKES 4 SERVINGS.

EASY SIDE SALADS

THE EATINGWELL DIET HOUSE SALAD

Starting a meal with a "garden" or "house" salad at restaurants is a winning appetite-cutting strategy that works just as well at home. This everyday side salad is a breeze to make; try it with soup or a sandwich for lunch, or for your first course at dinner.

4	cups torn green leaf lettuce
1	cup sprouts
1	cup tomato wedges
1	cup peeled, sliced cucumber
1	cup shredded carrots
½	cup chopped radishes
½	cup Sesame Tamari Vinaigrette (*page 126*) or EatingWell Diet dressing of choice (*pages 125-127*)

Toss lettuce, sprouts, tomato, cucumber, carrots and radishes in a large bowl with the dressing until the vegetables are coated.

MAKES **4** SERVINGS, **1** ½ CUPS EACH.

PER SERVING:

71 CALORIES

3 g fat (0 g sat, 1 g mono)

0 mg cholesterol

11 g carbohydrate

2 g protein

3 g fiber

334 mg sodium

428 mg potassium

NUTRITION BONUS:
Vitamin A (140% daily value)
Vitamin C (30% dv)
Folate (16% dv)

Healthy ⚖ Weight

Lower ⬇ Carbs

ACTIVE TIME: **10 MINUTES**

TOTAL: **10 MINUTES**

Basic Green Salad with Vinaigrette

Whisk together 3 tablespoons extra-virgin olive oil, 2 tablespoons red-wine vinegar, 1 tablespoon chopped flat-leaf parsley and ½ teaspoon each finely chopped garlic and Dijon mustard. Season with salt and freshly ground pepper. Toss with 8 cups mixed salad greens.
MAKES **4** SERVINGS.
PER SERVING: **115 calories;** 11 g fat (2 g sat, 8 g mono); 0 mg cholesterol; 4 g carbohydrate; 2 g protein; 2 g fiber; 190 mg sodium; 356 mg potassium.
NUTRITION BONUS: Vitamin A (60% daily value), Folate (32% dv), Vitamin C (30% dv).

Black-Eyed Pea & Artichoke Salad

Thaw a 9-ounce package of frozen artichoke hearts. Cut each artichoke in half. Combine with two 15-ounce cans of black-eyed peas, rinsed, ½ cup chopped red onion, 2 tablespoons balsamic vinegar, 1 ½ table-spoons extra-virgin olive oil, 1 teaspoon Worcester-shire sauce and ½ teaspoon caraway seeds. Season with salt and freshly ground pepper.
MAKES **6** SERVINGS.
PER SERVING: **167 calories;** 5 g fat (1 g sat, 3 g mono); 0 mg cholesterol; 25 g carbohydrate; 8 g protein; 7 g fiber; 356 mg sodium; 379 mg potassium.
NUTRITION BONUS: Folate (30% daily value).

Chickpea Salad

Rinse one 7-ounce can chickpeas and place in a medium bowl. Add 3 cups peeled, seeded and diced cucumber, 2 cups halved grape tomatoes (or cherry tomatoes), ¼ cup crumbled reduced-fat feta cheese, ¼ cup diced red onion, ½ cup EatingWell Diet dressing, such as Creamy Dill Ranch (*page 126*) and freshly ground pepper to taste. Mix until coated.

MAKES 6 SERVINGS, 1 CUP EACH.

PER SERVING: 90 calories; 2 g fat (1 g sat, 0 g mono); 3 mg cholesterol; 14 g carbohydrate; 5 g protein; 3 g fiber; 238 mg sodium; 285 mg potassium. NUTRITION BONUS: Vitamin C (15% daily value).

Chopped Tomato Salad

Chop 4 large tomatoes and combine with ¼ cup chopped fresh basil, 1 tablespoon extra-virgin olive oil and 1 teaspoon lemon juice. Season with salt and freshly ground pepper just before serving.

MAKES 4 SERVINGS.

PER SERVING: 65 calories; 4 g fat (1 g sat, 3 g mono); 0 mg cholesterol; 7 g carbohydrate; 2 g protein; 2 g fiber; 9 mg sodium; 445 mg potassium. NUTRITION BONUS: Vitamin C (40% daily value), Vitamin A (35% dv).

Cucumber Salad

Whisk together 1 tablespoon rice-wine vinegar, ¼ teaspoon sugar and a pinch of cayenne pepper. Season with salt and freshly ground pepper. Peel 2 cucumbers, halve lengthwise and seed; cut into ¼-inch thick slices. Toss with the dressing. Chill until ready to serve.

MAKES 4 SERVINGS.

PER SERVING: 24 calories; 0 g fat (0 g sat, 0 g mono); 0 mg cholesterol; 6 g carbohydrate; 1 g protein; 1 g fiber; 148 mg sodium; 222 mg potassium.

Endive & Watercress Salad

Trim 2 heads of Belgian endive. Break leaves into 1½-inch lengths. Thinly slice ½ small red onion. Whisk together 2 tablespoons apple cider, 1 tablespoon each extra-virgin olive oil and white-wine vinegar, and salt and freshly ground pepper to taste. Toss with 2 cups watercress leaves, the endive and the red onion.

MAKES 4 SERVINGS.

PER SERVING: 46 calories; 4 g fat (1 g sat, 3 g mono); 0 mg cholesterol; 3 g carbohydrate; 1 g protein; 1 g fiber; 0 mg sodium; 78 mg potassium. NUTRITION BONUS: Vitamin A & Vitamin C (15% daily value).

Greens with Parmesan Vinaigrette

Whisk together ⅓ cup freshly grated Parmesan cheese, 3 tablespoons extra-virgin olive oil, 2 tablespoons white-wine vinegar, ½ teaspoon minced garlic and ½ teaspoon Dijon mustard. Season with salt and freshly ground pepper. Toss with 8 cups mixed salad greens.

MAKES 4 SERVINGS.

PER SERVING: 154 calories; 13 g fat (3 g sat, 8 g mono); 7 mg cholesterol; 3 g carbohydrate; 6 g protein; 2 g fiber; 275 mg sodium; 350 mg potassium. NUTRITION BONUS: Vitamin A (60% daily value), Folate (32% dv), Vitamin C (30% dv), Calcium (20% dv).

Lemony Carrot Salad

Whisk 2 tablespoons each lemon juice and extra-virgin olive oil, 1 small minced garlic clove, ¼ teaspoon salt and freshly ground pepper to taste in a medium bowl. Add 2 cups grated carrots, 3 tablespoons chopped fresh dill and 2 tablespoons chopped scallion; toss to coat.

MAKES 4 SERVINGS, ½ CUP EACH.

PER SERVING: 90 calories; 7 g fat (1 g sat, 5 g mono); 0 mg cholesterol; 6 g carbohydrate; 1 g protein; 2 g fiber; 184 mg sodium; 198 mg potassium. NUTRITION BONUS: Vitamin A (130% daily value), Vitamin C (15% dv).

Napa Cabbage Slaw

Shred 8 ounces each napa cabbage, peeled carrots and peeled jícama using the large-hole side of a box grater. Mix with ¼ cup low-fat creamy salad dressing and 1 tablespoon Dijon mustard. Season with salt and freshly ground pepper.

MAKES 4 SERVINGS.

PER SERVING: 93 calories; 3 g fat (1 g sat, 0 g mono); 4 mg cholesterol; 14 g carbohydrate; 2 g protein; 5 g fiber; 374 mg sodium; 270 mg potassium. NUTRITION BONUS: Vitamin A (210% daily value), Vitamin C (50% dv).

Rainbow Chopped Salad

Place 1½ cups chopped bell peppers, 1½ cups chopped broccoli florets, 1 cup shredded carrots, ½ cup diced radishes, ½ cup Orange-Oregano Dressing (*page 127*) or Creamy Dill Ranch Dressing (*page 126*) and 1 tablespoon minced red onion in a medium bowl. Toss to coat. Refrigerate until ready to serve.

MAKES 4 SERVINGS, GENEROUS 1 CUP EACH.
PER SERVING: 64 calories; 2 g fat (0 g sat, 1 g mono); 0 mg cholesterol; 10 g carbohydrate; 2 g protein; 3 g fiber; 198 mg sodium; 371 mg potassium.
NUTRITION BONUS: Vitamin C (240% daily value), Vitamin A (140% dv).

Sliced Tomato Salad

Slice 4 tomatoes; arrange on a platter. Top with thinly sliced red onion, anchovies, dried oregano, salt and freshly ground pepper. Drizzle with 2 tablespoons extra-virgin olive oil and 1 tablespoon white-wine vinegar.

MAKES 4 SERVINGS.
PER SERVING: 44 calories; 1 g fat (0 g sat, 0 g mono); 3 mg cholesterol; 8 g carbohydrate; 3 g protein; 2 g fiber; 300 mg sodium; 403 mg potassium.
NUTRITION BONUS: Vitamin C (35% daily value), Vitamin A (25% dv).

Vinegary Coleslaw

Whisk ¼ cup white-wine vinegar, 2 tablespoons canola oil, 2 teaspoons each sugar and Dijon mustard, and ¼ teaspoon each of celery seed and salt in a medium bowl. Add 3 cups shredded cabbage, 2 grated carrots and ½ cup slivered red onion and toss to coat.

MAKES 4 SERVINGS, ABOUT 1 CUP EACH.
PER SERVING: 101 calories; 7 g fat (1 g sat, 4 g mono); 0 mg cholesterol; 9 g carbohydrate; 1 g protein; 2 g fiber; 138 mg sodium; 248 mg potassium.
NUTRITION BONUS: Vitamin A (100% daily value).

Warm Apple-Cabbage Salad

Place 3 cups shredded cabbage, 2 thinly sliced apples and ½ cup apple juice (*or* broth *or* water) in a large skillet, cover and cook until tender. Stir in cider vinegar and salt to taste.

MAKES 4 SERVINGS.

PER SERVING: 68 calories; 0 g fat (0 g sat, 0 g mono); 0 mg cholesterol; 18 g carbohydrate; 1 g protein; 4 g fiber; 156 mg sodium; 168 mg potassium.
NUTRITION BONUS: Vitamin C (35% daily value).

Watercress Salad

Trim 2 bunches watercress. Whisk together 2 tablespoons each reduced-sodium soy sauce and white vinegar and 1 tablespoon sesame oil. Toss with watercress and season with freshly ground pepper.

MAKES 4 SERVINGS.
PER SERVING: 38 calories; 4 g fat (1 g sat, 2 g mono); 0 mg cholesterol; 1 g carbohydrate; 1 g protein; 0 g fiber; 281 mg sodium; 127 mg potassium.
NUTRITION BONUS: Vitamin A (30% daily value), Vitamin C (25% dv).

The Wedge

Quarter 2 hearts of romaine lengthwise; remove core. Top with 2 tablespoons chopped chives, 2 crumbled slices bacon and ¼ cup crumbled blue cheese. Top with Creamy Dill Ranch Dressing (*page 126*).

MAKES 4 SERVINGS.
PER SERVING: 70 calories; 5 g fat (2 g sat, 1 g mono); 11 mg cholesterol; 3 g carbohydrate; 4 g protein; 1 g fiber; 297 mg sodium; 61 mg potassium.
NUTRITION BONUS: Vitamin A (25% daily value).

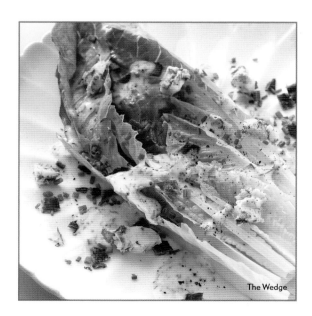
The Wedge

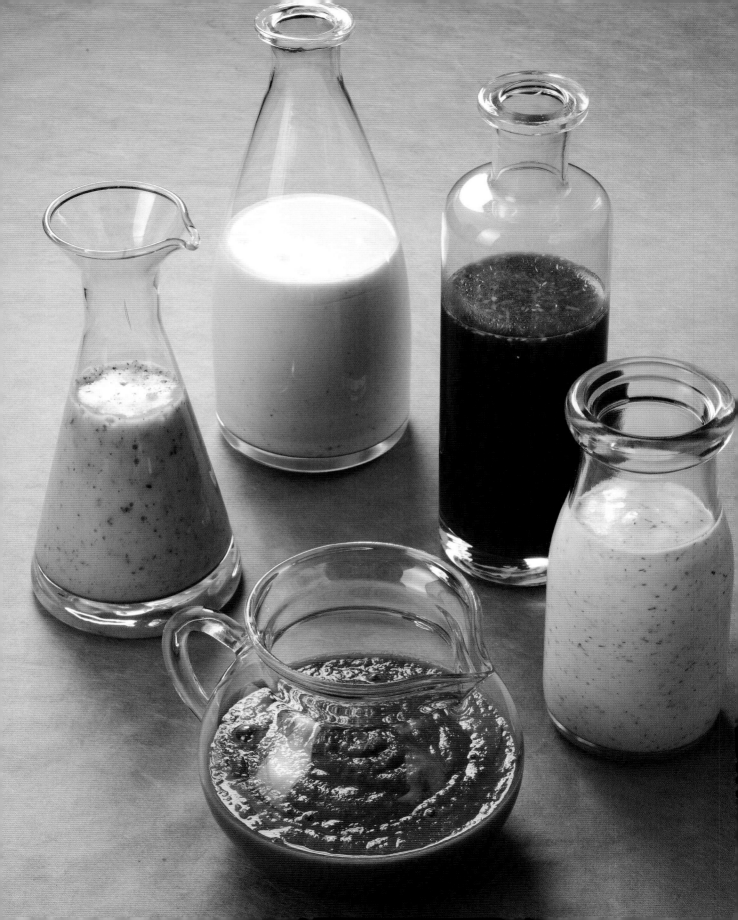

ROASTED TOMATO VINAIGRETTE

Invest a little extra time in this recipe to slow-roast the tomatoes and you're rewarded with a rich, earthy flavor with almost no fat.

12	ounces plum tomatoes, halved lengthwise and cored
1	tablespoon chopped garlic
1	tablespoon extra-virgin olive oil
1	teaspoon Italian seasoning mix
1	teaspoon kosher salt
	Freshly ground pepper to taste
2	tablespoons sherry vinegar *or* red-wine vinegar

1. Preheat oven to 300°F. Coat an 8-inch-square glass baking dish with cooking spray.

2. Toss tomatoes, garlic, oil, Italian seasoning, salt and pepper in a medium bowl. Spread the tomatoes in the prepared baking dish. Bake until the tomatoes are broken down and the juices are thick and syrupy, 1 hour 20 minutes to 1 hour 35 minutes.

3. Transfer the tomatoes to a blender. Add vinegar and puree. (Use caution when blending hot mixtures.) Cool completely before using.

MAKES 1 CUP.

PER **2-TABLESPOON SERVING:**

19 CALORIES

1 g fat (0 g sat, 1 g mono)
0 mg cholesterol
1 g carbohydrate
0 g protein
0 g fiber
99 mg sodium
59 mg potassium

ACTIVE TIME: **10 MINUTES**

TOTAL: **2 HOURS**

TO MAKE AHEAD: **Cover and refrigerate for up to 1 week. Stir before using.**

Opposite, clockwise from front: Roasted Tomato Vinaigrette, Orange-Oregano Dressing (*page 127*), Creamy Blue Cheese Dressing (*page 127*), Sesame Tamari Vinaigrette (*page 126*), Creamy Dill Ranch Dressing (*page 126*).

CREAMY DILL RANCH DRESSING

Cottage cheese blended in a food processor to a creamy texture, while not traditional in Ranch dressing, delivers unbelievable richness with minimal calories and fat.

1	small shallot, peeled
¾	cup nonfat cottage cheese
¼	cup reduced-fat mayonnaise
2	tablespoons buttermilk powder (*see Note, page 245*)
2	tablespoons white-wine vinegar
¼	cup nonfat milk
1	tablespoon chopped dill
¼	teaspoon salt
¼	teaspoon freshly ground pepper

With the food processor running, add shallot through the feed tube and process until finely chopped. Add cottage cheese, mayonnaise, buttermilk powder and vinegar. Process until smooth, scraping down the sides as necessary, about 3 minutes. Pour in milk while the processor is running. Scrape down the sides, add dill, salt and pepper and process until combined.

MAKES 1 ¼ CUPS.

SESAME TAMARI VINAIGRETTE

The roasted-nut and citrus flavors of this easy dressing go well with Asian-style salads or meals; try drizzling it on grilled shrimp or chicken breast, too.

¼	cup orange juice
¼	cup rice vinegar
2	tablespoons reduced-sodium tamari *or* reduced-sodium soy sauce
1	tablespoon toasted sesame oil
1	tablespoon honey
1	teaspoon finely grated fresh ginger

Whisk orange juice, vinegar, tamari, oil, honey and ginger in a small bowl until the honey is incorporated. Transfer to a jar and refrigerate.

MAKES ¾ CUP.

CREAMY BLUE CHEESE DRESSING

Creamy blue cheese dressing is still rich and delicious when you make it with low-fat dairy products and reduced-fat mayonnaise. Choose the tangiest aged blue cheese you can find; its flavor will go a long way.

- 1/3 cup reduced-fat mayonnaise
- 1/3 cup nonfat buttermilk *or* nonfat milk
- 1/3 cup nonfat plain yogurt
- 2 tablespoons tarragon vinegar *or* white vinegar
- 1 tablespoon Dijon mustard
- 1/2 teaspoon salt
- 1/2 teaspoon freshly ground pepper
- 1/4 cup crumbled blue cheese (1 ounce)

Whisk mayonnaise, buttermilk (or milk), yogurt, vinegar, mustard, salt and pepper in a medium bowl until smooth. Add cheese and stir, mashing with a spoon until the cheese is incorporated.

MAKES 1 1/4 CUPS.

PER 2-TABLESPOON SERVING:

38 CALORIES

3 g fat (1 g sat, 1 g mono)
4 mg cholesterol
2 g carbohydrate
1 g protein
0 g fiber
215 mg sodium
8 mg potassium

ACTIVE TIME: **10 MINUTES**

TOTAL: **10 MINUTES**

TO MAKE AHEAD: **Cover and refrigerate for up to 1 week. Stir before using.**

ORANGE-OREGANO DRESSING

What this dressing lacks in calories and fat it makes up for in big, bold orange flavor and herbal oregano notes.

- 1/2 teaspoon orange zest
- 1/2 cup orange juice, preferably freshly squeezed
- 1/4 cup cider vinegar
- 1 tablespoon extra-virgin olive oil
- 2 teaspoons chopped fresh oregano *or* 3/4 teaspoon dried
- 1 teaspoon Dijon mustard
- 1/2 teaspoon salt
- 1/2 teaspoon freshly ground pepper

Place all ingredients in a jar. Cover and shake to combine.

MAKES ABOUT 1 CUP.

PER 2-TABLESPOON SERVING:

27 CALORIES

2 g fat (0 g sat, 1 g mono)
0 mg cholesterol
2 g carbohydrate
0 g protein
0 g fiber
165 mg sodium
41 mg potassium

ACTIVE TIME: **5 MINUTES**

TOTAL: **5 MINUTES**

TO MAKE AHEAD: **Cover and refrigerate for up to 1 week.**

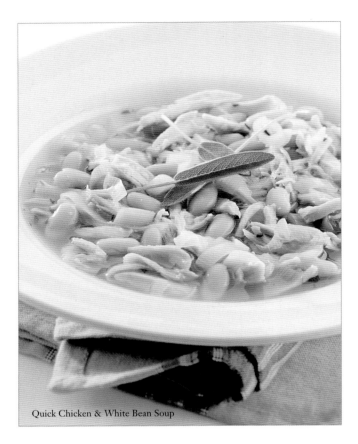

Quick Chicken & White Bean Soup

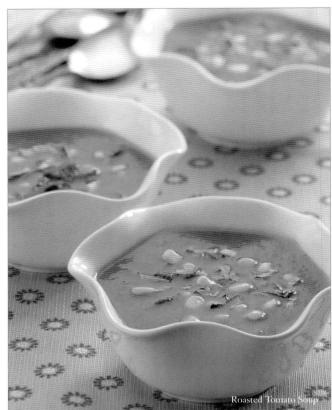

Roasted Tomato Soup

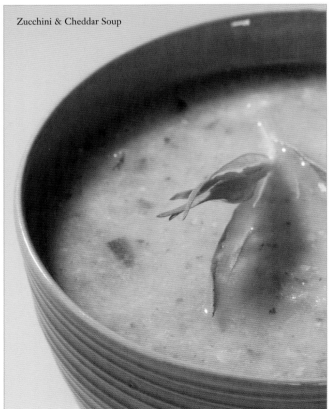

Zucchini & Cheddar Soup

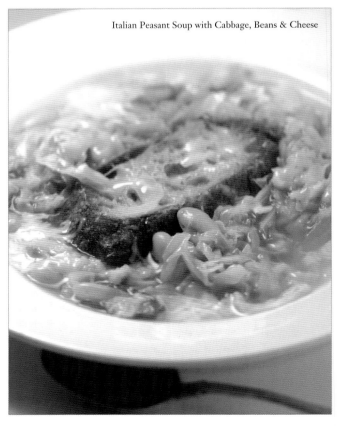

Italian Peasant Soup with Cabbage, Beans & Cheese

SOUPS

"To feel safe and warm on a cold wet night,
all you really need is soup. **"**

LAURIE COLWIN, AUTHOR & FOOD WRITER

191 CALORIES

4 g fat (2 g sat, 1 g mono)

64 mg cholesterol

14 g carbohydrate

24 g protein

1 g fiber

182 mg sodium

133 mg potassium

NUTRITION BONUS:
Vitamin A (50% daily value)

Healthy)(Weight

Lower ⬇ Carbs

ACTIVE TIME: **20 MINUTES**

TOTAL: **50 MINUTES**

TO MAKE AHEAD: **The soup will keep, covered, in the refrigerator for up to 2 days.**

CHICKEN NOODLE SOUP WITH DILL

This recipe for "Grandma's penicillin" has a long lineage. Passed from mother to daughter, friend to friend, on to EATINGWELL *recipe tester Deidre Senior, each cook has given the recipe her own touch, resulting in a superb healing antidote to any winter chill.*

10	cups chicken broth, homemade or reduced-sodium canned
3	medium carrots, peeled and diced
1	large stalk celery, diced
3	tablespoons minced fresh ginger
6	cloves garlic, minced
4	ounces dried egg noodles (3 cups)
4	cups shredded cooked skinless chicken (about 1 pound)
3	tablespoons chopped fresh dill
1	tablespoon lemon juice, or to taste

1. Bring broth to a boil in a Dutch oven. Add carrots, celery, ginger and garlic; cook, uncovered, over medium heat until vegetables are just tender, about 20 minutes.

2. Add noodles and chicken; continue cooking until the noodles are just tender, 8 to 10 minutes. Stir in dill and lemon juice.

MAKES **9** SERVINGS, ABOUT **1** CUP EACH.

ROASTED TOMATO SOUP

Roasting the vegetables for this simple summer soup enhances their inherent sweetness. The recipe is from EatingWell *reader Tracey Medeiros of Atlanta, Georgia.*

1½   pounds large tomatoes, such as beefsteak, cut in half crosswise
1   medium sweet onion, such as Vidalia, peeled and cut in half crosswise
3   large cloves garlic, unpeeled
1   tablespoon plus 1 teaspoon extra-virgin olive oil, divided
¼   teaspoon salt, or to taste
   Freshly ground pepper to taste
2   cups reduced-sodium chicken broth *or* vegetable broth, divided
¼   cup tomato juice
1   teaspoon tomato paste
¼   teaspoon Worcestershire sauce
1   tablespoon fresh basil, chopped
   Brown sugar to taste (optional)
½   cup corn kernels (fresh, from 1 ear; *see Tip*) *or* frozen, thawed

1. Preheat oven to 400°F. Coat a baking sheet with cooking spray.
2. Toss tomatoes, onion and garlic in a mixing bowl with 1 tablespoon oil. Season with salt and pepper. Spread on the prepared baking sheet and roast until the vegetables are soft and caramelized, about 30 minutes. Let cool.
3. Peel and seed the tomatoes. Trim off the onion ends. Peel the garlic. Place the vegetables in a food processor or blender with 1 cup broth and the remaining 1 teaspoon oil. Pulse to desired thickness and texture.
4. Transfer the vegetable puree to a large heavy pot or Dutch oven. Add the remaining 1 cup broth, tomato juice, tomato paste, Worcestershire sauce, basil and brown sugar (if using). Bring to a simmer over medium heat, stirring often. Ladle into 6 soup bowls, garnish with corn and serve.

MAKES 6 SERVINGS, 1 CUP EACH.

PER SERVING:

95 CALORIES

4 g fat (1 g sat, 3 g mono)
1 mg cholesterol
13 g carbohydrate
3 g protein
3 g fiber
146 mg sodium
406 mg potassium

NUTRITION BONUS:
Vitamin C (35% daily value)
Vitamin A (20% dv)

Healthy ⅓ Weight

Lower ⬇ Carbs

ACTIVE TIME: **35 MINUTES**

TOTAL: **45 MINUTES**

TO MAKE AHEAD: **Cover and refrigerate for up to 2 days or freeze for up to 2 months.**

TIP

- To remove corn from the cob, stand an uncooked ear of corn on its stem end in a shallow bowl and slice the kernels off with a sharp, thin-bladed knife.

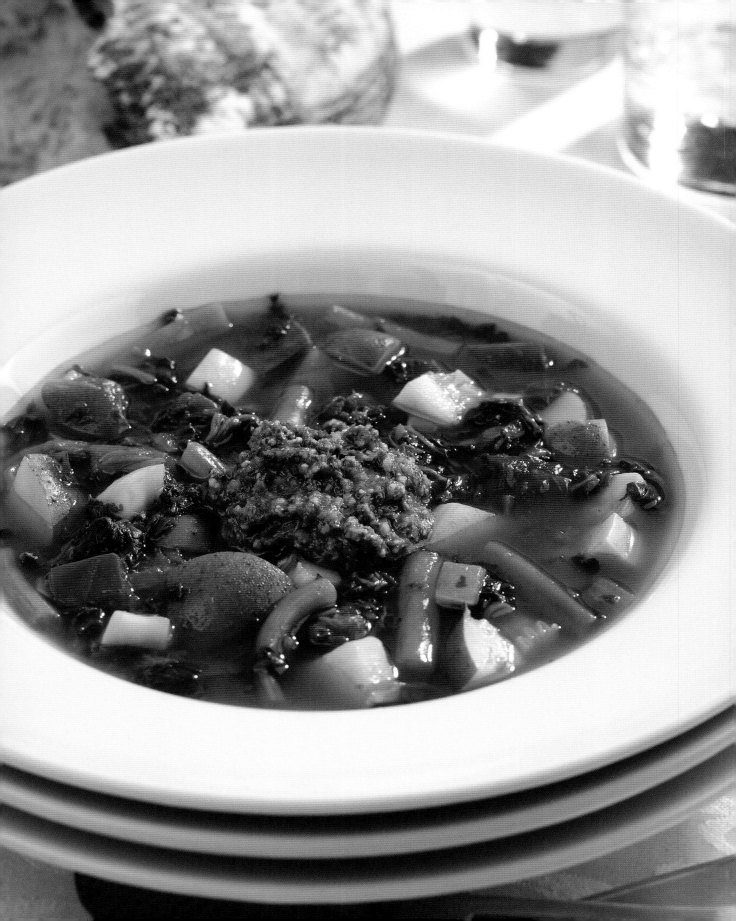

SPICY VEGETABLE SOUP

Getting three-plus servings of vegetables has never been easier. Here, they're combined with the traditional flavors of the Mediterranean—tangy sherry vinegar, earthy paprika and fragrant basil—to make a soul-satisfying soup that tastes even better a day later. Using pesto instead of fresh basil adds nutty richness.

2	tablespoons extra-virgin olive oil
1	large onion, diced
1-3	teaspoons hot paprika, or to taste
2	14-ounce cans vegetable broth
4	medium plum tomatoes, diced
1	medium yellow summer squash, diced
2	cups diced cooked potatoes (*see Ingredient Note, page 245*)
1½	cups green beans, cut into 2-inch pieces
2	cups frozen spinach (5 ounces)
2	tablespoons sherry vinegar *or* red-wine vinegar
¼	cup chopped fresh basil *or* prepared pesto

Heat oil in a Dutch oven over medium heat. Add onion, cover and cook, stirring occasionally, until beginning to brown, about 6 minutes. Add paprika and cook, stirring, for 30 seconds. Add broth, tomatoes, squash, potatoes and beans; bring to a boil. Reduce heat to a simmer and cook, stirring occasionally, until the vegetables are just tender, about 12 minutes. Stir in spinach and vinegar; continue cooking until heated through, 2 to 4 minutes more. Ladle soup into bowls and top with fresh basil or a dollop of pesto.

MAKES **4** SERVINGS, ABOUT **2 ¼** CUPS EACH.

PER SERVING:

253 CALORIES

8 g fat (1 g sat, 5 g mono)

0 mg cholesterol

40 g carbohydrate

9 g protein

10 g fiber

485 mg sodium

1,032 mg potassium

NUTRITION BONUS:
Vitamin A (270% daily value)
Vitamin C (60% dv)
Folate (44% dv)
Potassium (30% dv)
Calcium & Iron (20% dv)

High ⬆ Fiber

ACTIVE TIME: **30 MINUTES**

TOTAL: **40 MINUTES**

TO MAKE AHEAD: **Cover and refrigerate for up to 2 days.**

241 CALORIES

3 g fat (1 g sat, 1 g mono)

33 mg cholesterol

32 g carbohydrate

25 g protein

5 g fiber

370 mg sodium

617 mg potassium

NUTRITION BONUS:
Vitamin A (260% daily value)
Vitamin C (120% dv)
Folate (21% dv)
Iron (20% dv)

Healthy ⅓ Weight

High ⬆ Fiber

ACTIVE TIME: **35 MINUTES**

TOTAL: **45 MINUTES**

HEARTY TURKEY & SQUASH SOUP

Full of fall flavors, this soup is a meal in a bowl. You can also make it with diced cooked turkey (or chicken), adding it near the end and simmering it a few minutes extra, just until the meat is firm and opaque.

2	teaspoons canola oil
2	leeks, trimmed, thoroughly cleaned and chopped (3½ cups)
1	red bell pepper, seeded and chopped
3	cloves garlic, finely chopped
4	cups reduced-sodium chicken broth
1½	pounds butternut squash (2 medium), peeled, seeded and cut into 1-inch cubes
2	tablespoons chopped fresh thyme *or* 2 teaspoons dried thyme leaves
1½	teaspoons ground cumin
1	pound turkey cutlets, cut into ½-by-2-inch strips
2	cups frozen corn kernels
2	tablespoons lime juice
½	teaspoon crushed red pepper
	Salt & freshly ground pepper to taste

1. Heat oil in a large heavy pot over medium-high heat. Add leeks and pepper; cook, stirring often, until the vegetables begin to soften, 3 to 4 minutes. Add garlic and cook, stirring constantly, 1 minute more.

2. Stir in broth, squash, thyme and cumin; cover and bring to a boil. Reduce heat to medium-low and cook until the vegetables are tender, about 10 minutes.

3. Add turkey and corn; return the broth to a simmer. Simmer until the turkey is just cooked through, 3 to 4 minutes. Add lime juice and crushed red pepper. Gently warm the soup until heated through. Season with salt and pepper.

MAKES **6** SERVINGS, ABOUT **1½** CUPS EACH.

ITALIAN PEASANT SOUP WITH CABBAGE, BEANS & CHEESE

This hearty, fiber-packed soup has slow-cooked flavor, but comes together quickly with a few pantry staples.

2   19-ounce *or* 15 1/2-ounce cans cannellini beans, rinsed, divided
3   tablespoons extra-virgin olive oil, divided
1   medium onion, halved and sliced
4   cups shredded Savoy cabbage (1/2 medium head)
3   cloves garlic, minced, plus 1 clove garlic, halved
3   14 1/2-ounce cans reduced-sodium chicken broth *or* 5 1/4 cups
     vegetable broth
     Freshly ground pepper to taste
8   1/2-inch-thick slices day-old whole-wheat country bread
1   cup grated fontina cheese *or* 1/2 cup Parmesan cheese

1. Mash 1 1/2 cups beans with a fork.
2. Heat 1 teaspoon oil over medium heat in a Dutch oven or soup pot. Add onion and cook, stirring often, until softened and lightly browned, 2 to 3 minutes. Add cabbage and minced garlic; cook, stirring often, until the cabbage has wilted, 2 to 3 minutes. Add broth, mashed beans and whole beans; bring to a simmer. Reduce heat to medium-low, partially cover and simmer until the cabbage is tender, 10 to 12 minutes. Season with pepper.
3. Shortly before the soup is ready, toast bread lightly and rub with the cut side of the garlic clove (lightly or heavily depending on taste). Divide toast among 8 soup plates. Ladle soup over the toast and sprinkle with cheese. Drizzle about 1 teaspoon oil over each serving. Serve immediately.

MAKES 8 SERVINGS, 1 CUP EACH.

PER SERVING:

303 CALORIES

12 g fat (4 g sat, 5 g mono)
18 mg cholesterol
38 g carbohydrate
14 g protein
12 g fiber
552 mg sodium
124 mg potassium

NUTRITION BONUS:
Fiber (47% daily value)
Calcium (25% dv)
Folate (17% dv)

Healthy)(Weight

High ⬆ Fiber

ACTIVE TIME: **30 MINUTES**

TOTAL: **40 MINUTES**

TO MAKE AHEAD: **Prepare through Step 2. Cover and refrigerate for up to 2 days. Reheat on the stovetop and continue with Step 3.**

199 CALORIES

6 g fat (1 g sat, 3 g mono)

52 mg cholesterol

16 g carbohydrate

23 g protein

4 g fiber

530 mg sodium

233 mg potassium

NUTRITION BONUS:
Selenium (19% daily value)
Iron (15% dv)

Healthy ⋊ Weight

Lower ⬇ Carbs

ACTIVE TIME: **25 MINUTES**

TOTAL: **25 MINUTES**

TO MAKE AHEAD: **Cover and refrigerate for up to 2 days.**

QUICK CHICKEN & WHITE BEAN SOUP

Available in just about every supermarket these days, rotisserie chickens can really relieve the dinner-rush pressure. The soup needs just a brief simmer; add a little crusty whole-grain bread and you've got dinner in 10 minutes flat.

- 2 teaspoons extra-virgin olive oil
- 2 leeks, white and light green parts only, cut into ¼-inch rounds
- 1 tablespoon chopped fresh sage *or* ¼ teaspoon dried
- 2 14-ounce cans reduced-sodium chicken broth
- 2 cups water
- 1 15-ounce can cannellini beans, rinsed
- 1 2-pound roasted chicken, skin discarded, meat removed from bones and shredded (4 cups)

Heat oil in a Dutch oven over medium-high heat. Add leeks and cook, stirring often, until soft, about 3 minutes. Stir in sage and continue cooking until aromatic, about 30 seconds. Stir in broth and water, increase heat to high, cover and bring to a boil. Add beans and chicken and cook, uncovered, stirring occasionally, until heated through, about 3 minutes. Serve hot.

MAKES **6** SERVINGS, 1 ½ CUPS EACH.

CHICKEN TORTILLA SOUP

A few simple fresh ingredients—plus a few choice convenience products—make this Tex-Mex favorite as simple as it is delicious. Why not make a double batch of the tortilla strips to sprinkle on salads, stews and other soups?

4	soft corn tortillas, cut into 1-by-2-inch strips
1	tablespoon extra-virgin olive oil
1	pound boneless, skinless chicken breast, trimmed of fat and diced
3	cups frozen bell pepper and onion mix (about 10 ounces)
1	tablespoon ground cumin
2	14-ounce cans reduced-sodium chicken broth
1	15-ounce can diced tomatoes, preferably with green chiles
¼	teaspoon freshly ground pepper
2	tablespoons lime juice
½	cup chopped fresh cilantro
¾	cup shredded reduced-fat Cheddar *or* Monterey Jack cheese

1. Preheat oven to 350°F. Spread tortillas in a single layer on a baking sheet. Bake until lightly browned and crisp, 10 to 12 minutes.

2. Meanwhile, heat oil in a Dutch oven over medium-high heat. Add chicken and cook, stirring occasionally, until beginning to brown, 3 to 4 minutes. Transfer to a plate using a slotted spoon. Add pepper-onion mix and cumin to the pot. Cook, stirring occasionally, until the onions are lightly browned, about 4 minutes. Add broth, tomatoes, pepper and lime juice; bring to a simmer and cook, stirring often, until the vegetables are tender, about 3 minutes more. Return the chicken and any accumulated juice to the pot and cook, stirring, until heated through, about 1 minute. Remove from the heat; stir in cilantro. Serve topped with the toasted tortilla strips and cheese.

MAKES 4 SERVINGS, ABOUT 1 1/3 CUPS EACH.

PER SERVING:

357 CALORIES

12 g fat (5 g sat, 4 g mono)
87 mg cholesterol
24 g carbohydrate
37 g protein
4 g fiber
603 mg sodium
231 mg potassium

NUTRITION BONUS:
Selenium (30% daily value)
Calcium (20% dv)
Vitamin C & Zinc (15% dv)

ACTIVE TIME: **35 MINUTES**

TOTAL: **35 MINUTES**

TO MAKE AHEAD: **Cover and refrigerate, without the tortilla strips, for up to 2 days. Top with toasted tortilla strips just before serving.**

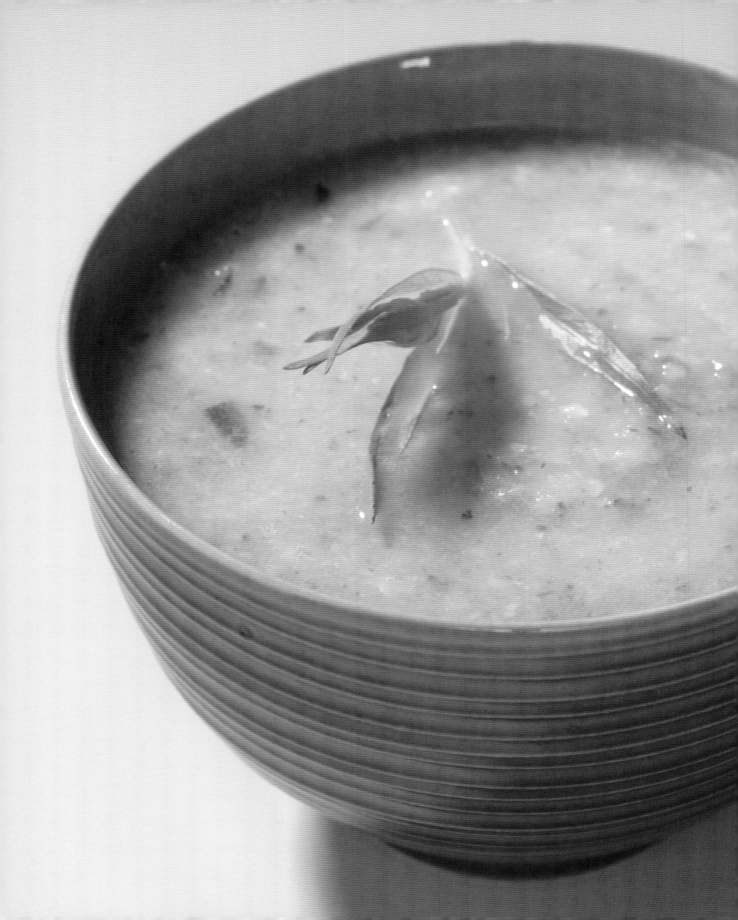

ZUCCHINI & CHEDDAR SOUP

This is one of the few soups that make the cut in summer. Serve it chilled to take the edge off a hot August night.

3	cups reduced-sodium chicken broth
1 ½	pounds zucchini (about 3 medium), cut into 1-inch pieces
1	tablespoon chopped fresh tarragon *or* dill *or* 1 teaspoon dried
¾	cup shredded reduced-fat Cheddar cheese (3 ounces)
¼	teaspoon salt
¼	teaspoon freshly ground pepper

Place broth, zucchini and tarragon (or dill) in a medium saucepan; bring to a boil over high heat. Reduce to a simmer and cook, uncovered, until the zucchini is tender, 7 to 10 minutes. Puree in a blender, in batches if necessary, until smooth. Return the soup to the pan and heat over medium-high heat, slowly stirring in cheese until it is incorporated. Remove from heat and season with salt and pepper. Serve hot or chilled.

MAKES 4 SERVINGS, 1 ¼ CUPS EACH.

PER SERVING:

115 CALORIES

5 g fat (3 g sat, 0 g mono)
19 mg cholesterol
7 g carbohydrate
10 g protein
2 g fiber
448 mg sodium
452 mg potassium

NUTRITION BONUS:
Vitamin C (50% daily value)
Calcium (20% dv)

Healthy)((Weight

Lower ⬇ Carbs

ACTIVE TIME: **15 MINUTES**

TOTAL: **20 MINUTES**

TO MAKE AHEAD: **Cover and refrigerate for up to 3 days. Serve chilled or reheat.**

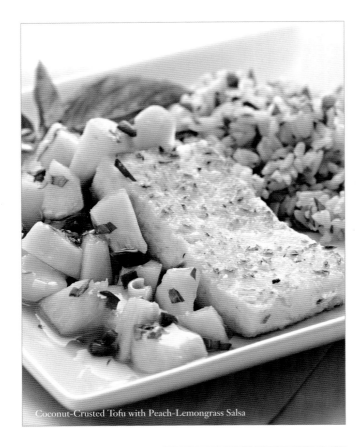

Coconut-Crusted Tofu with Peach-Lemongrass Salsa

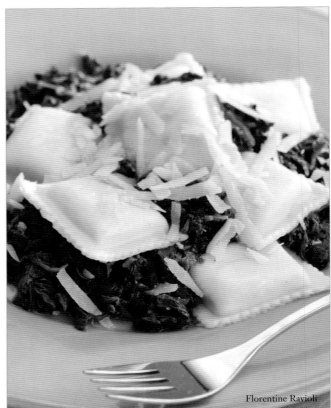

Florentine Ravioli

Peanut-Ginger Tofu & Vegetables

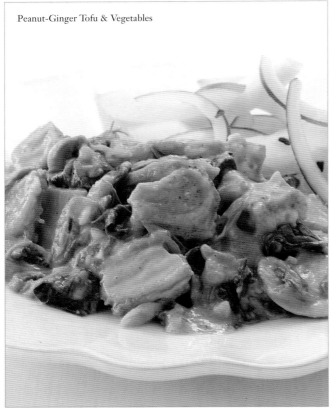

Mediterranean Portobello Burger

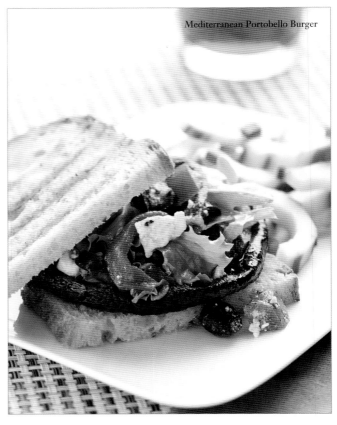

VEGETARIAN

❝ The more you eat, the less flavor;
the less you eat, the more flavor. **❞**

CHINESE PROVERB

ACTIVE TIME: **30 MINUTES**

TOTAL: **30 MINUTES**

MEDITERRANEAN PORTOBELLO BURGER

Grilled meaty portobello mushrooms make a hearty vegetarian sandwich that's as good as a burger anytime. Layering the bread with Greek-style salad adds luscious flavor and textures—and a full serving of vegetables.

1	clove garlic, minced
1/2	teaspoon kosher salt
2	tablespoons extra-virgin olive oil, divided
4	portobello mushroom caps, stems and gills removed
4	large slices country-style sourdough bread, cut in half
1/2	cup sliced jarred roasted red peppers
1/2	cup chopped tomato
1/4	cup crumbled reduced-fat feta cheese
2	tablespoons chopped pitted Kalamata olives
1	tablespoon red-wine vinegar
1/2	teaspoon dried oregano
2	cups loosely packed mixed baby salad greens

1. Preheat grill to medium-high.

2. Mash garlic and salt on a cutting board with the side of a knife into a smooth paste. Mix the paste with 1 tablespoon oil in a small dish. Lightly brush the oil mixture over portobellos and then on one side of each slice of bread.

3. Combine red peppers, tomato, feta, olives, vinegar, oregano and the remaining 1 tablespoon oil in a medium bowl.

4. Grill the mushroom caps until tender, about 4 minutes per side; grill the bread until crisp, about 1 minute per side.

5. Toss salad greens with the red pepper mixture. Place the grilled mushrooms top-side down on 4 half-slices of the bread. Top with the salad mixture and the remaining bread.

MAKES 4 SERVINGS.

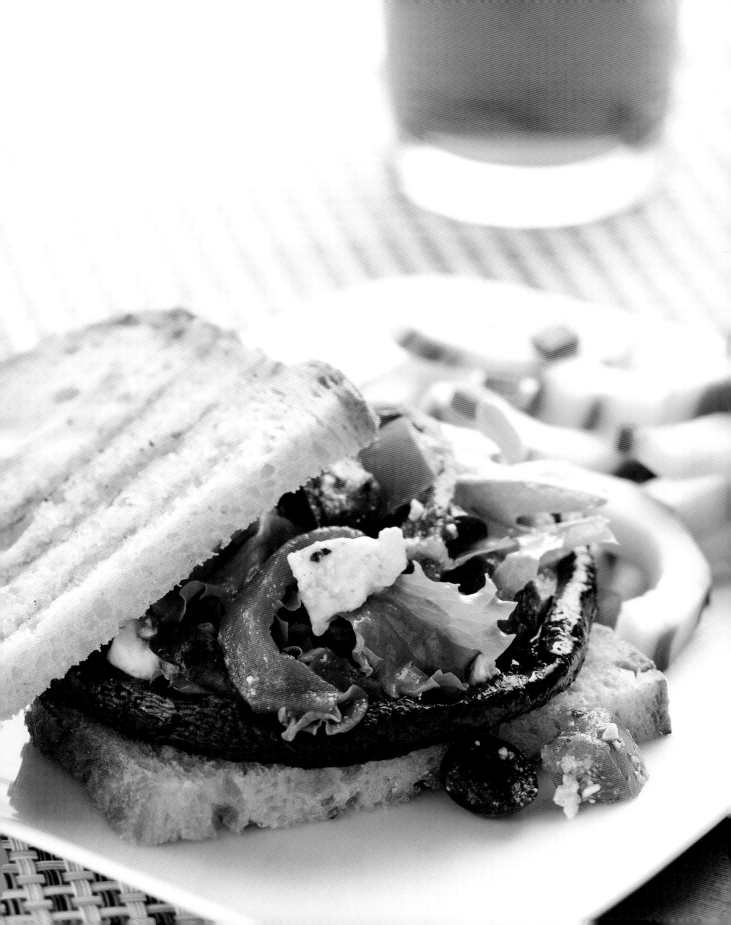

COOKING TIP:

■ The dark gills found on the underside of the mushroom are edible, but can turn food an unappealing gray/black color. Remove the gills with a spoon, if desired.

PORTOBELLO "PHILLY CHEESE STEAK" SANDWICH

Cheese steaks are a Philadelphia tradition: thin slices from a rich and very fatty slab of beef, fried up and topped with a heavy cheese sauce. We've made it vegetarian and cut down on the fat considerably—but not on the taste.

4	whole-wheat buns, split in half
2	teaspoons extra-virgin olive oil
1	medium onion, sliced
4	large portobello mushrooms, stems and gills removed (*see Tip*), sliced
1	large red bell pepper, thinly sliced
2	tablespoons minced fresh oregano *or* 2 teaspoons dried
1/2	teaspoon freshly ground pepper
1	tablespoon all-purpose flour
1/4	cup vegetable broth *or* reduced-sodium chicken broth
1	tablespoon reduced-sodium soy sauce
3	ounces thinly sliced reduced-fat provolone cheese

1. Toast buns in a toaster or in a 350°F oven.

2. Meanwhile, heat oil in a large nonstick skillet over medium-high heat. Add onion and cook, stirring often, until soft and beginning to brown, 2 to 3 minutes. Add mushrooms, bell pepper, oregano and pepper and cook, stirring often, until the vegetables are wilted and soft, about 7 minutes. Reduce heat to low; sprinkle the vegetables with flour and stir to coat. Stir in broth and soy sauce. Remove from the heat, lay cheese slices on top of the vegetables, cover and let stand until melted, 1 to 2 minutes. Divide the mixture into 4 portions with a spatula, leaving the melted cheese layer on top. Scoop a portion onto the bottom half of each toasted bun and serve immediately.

MAKES 4 SANDWICHES.

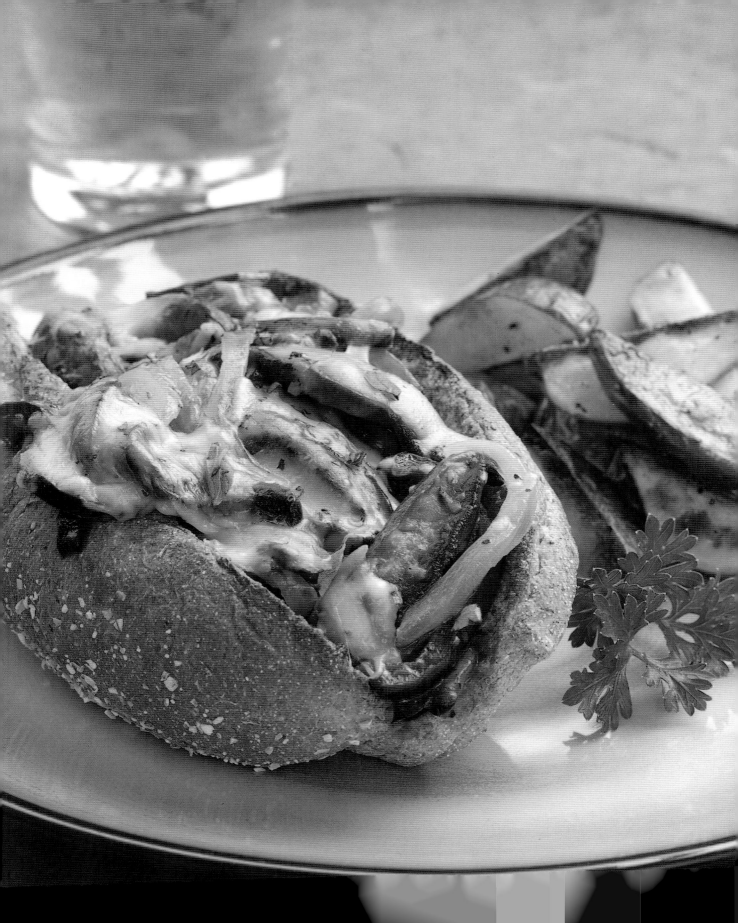

221 CALORIES

15 g fat (5 g sat, 3 g mono)

13 mg cholesterol

16 g carbohydrate

7 g protein

1 g fiber

429 mg sodium

59 mg potassium

NUTRITION BONUS:
Vitamin A (50% daily value)

Healthy)((Weight

Lower ⬇ Carbs

ACTIVE TIME: **15 MINUTES**

TOTAL: **15 MINUTES**

TO MAKE AHEAD: **Wrap in plastic wrap and store in the refrigerator or in a cooler with a cold pack for up to 8 hours.**

ROASTED RED PEPPER SUBS

When the occasion calls for a sophisticated sandwich, simply layer roasted red peppers, goat cheese and peppery arugula on a crusty baguette.

1	12-ounce jar roasted red peppers, rinsed
1	clove garlic, minced
1	tablespoon red-wine vinegar
1	teaspoon extra-virgin olive oil
	Pinch of salt
	Freshly ground pepper to taste
1	16- to 20-inch baguette, preferably whole-wheat
3	tablespoon olive paste (*olivada*)
4	ounces creamy goat cheese
1 ½	cups arugula leaves

1. Combine peppers, garlic, vinegar and oil in a small bowl; toss to combine. Season with salt and pepper.

2. Slice baguette in half lengthwise. Spread one half with olive paste and the other half with goat cheese. Layer pepper mixture and arugula over olive paste. Top with remaining baguette. Cut across into 4 pieces.

MAKES **4** SANDWICHES.

BUTTER-BEAN SPREAD ROLL-UP SANDWICH

This vegetarian sandwich is full of flavors and textures, and beans make it extra satisfying. We love the combination of onion, lettuce, fennel, carrot and sprouts, but equal amounts of whatever vegetables you like or have on hand will also work well.

1/4	cup Butter-Bean Spread (*recipe follows*)
1	whole-wheat lavash (*see Note, page 245*)
1	small slice red onion
1	cup torn lettuce
1/4	cup thinly sliced fennel
1/4	cup shredded carrot
1/4	cup mung bean sprouts

Spread butter-bean spread over the lavash, leaving a 1-inch border on the short sides. Arrange onion, lettuce, fennel, carrot and sprouts over the spread along one short side. Roll up and cut in half.

MAKES **1** SERVING.

BUTTER-BEAN SPREAD

Spread this bean puree on crackers, on a vegetable sandwich or dip assorted vegetables in it.

1	16-ounce can butter beans, drained and rinsed
1	scallion, sliced
1	small clove garlic, chopped
1/2	cup nonfat plain yogurt
1/4	cup grated Parmesan cheese
1	tablespoon extra-virgin olive oil
1	tablespoon red-wine vinegar
1/2	teaspoon chopped fresh rosemary *or* 1/4 teaspoon dried
1/4	teaspoon salt
1/4	teaspoon freshly ground pepper

Puree butter beans, scallion, garlic, yogurt, Parmesan, oil, vinegar, rosemary, salt and pepper in a food processor until smooth.

MAKES 1 2/3 CUPS.

PER SERVING:

343 CALORIES

3 g fat (1 g sat, 2 g mono)
3 mg cholesterol
62 g carbohydrate
15 g protein
13 g fiber
524 mg sodium
563 mg potassium

NUTRITION BONUS:
Vitamin A (130% daily value)
Vitamin C (20% dv)
Folate (18% dv)
Potassium (16% dv)

Healthy ⚖ Weight

High ⬆ Fiber

ACTIVE TIME: **15 MINUTES**

TOTAL: **15 MINUTES**

BUTTER-BEAN SPREAD
PER **2** TABLESPOONS:

35 CALORIES

2 g fat (0 g sat, 1 g mono)
2 mg cholesterol
5 g carbohydrate
2 g protein
1 g fiber
132 mg sodium
102 mg potassium

ACTIVE TIME: **10 MINUTES**

TOTAL: **10 MINUTES**

TO MAKE AHEAD: **Cover and refrigerate for up to 4 days.**

PER SERVING:

289 CALORIES

11 g fat (3 g sat, 4 g mono)

373 mg cholesterol

29 g carbohydrate

17 g protein

4 g fiber

600 mg sodium

289 mg potassium

NUTRITION BONUS:
Folate (30% daily value)
Vitamin A (20% dv)
Iron (15% dv)

Healthy ⚥ Weight

ACTIVE TIME: **10 MINUTES**

TOTAL: **10 MINUTES**

EGG SALAD SANDWICHES WITH WATERCRESS

Watercress, a cruciferous vegetable, adds a zesty note—and welcome phytonutrients—to this enlightened version of an American classic.

8   hard-boiled eggs (*see Tip, page 245*)
3   tablespoons nonfat sour cream *or* nonfat plain yogurt
1   tablespoon reduced-fat mayonnaise
1   tablespoon grainy mustard
4   scallions, trimmed and chopped
    Salt & freshly ground pepper to taste
¾   cup washed and stemmed watercress
8   slices pumpernickel bread

1. Scoop out egg yolks. Place 2 yolks in a small bowl and reserve the rest for another use. Chop egg whites and reserve. Mash the yolks with a fork and stir in sour cream (or yogurt), mayonnaise and mustard. Add chopped egg whites and scallions and season with salt and pepper.
2. Arrange watercress on 4 bread slices. Top with the egg salad and cover with the remaining bread slices.

MAKES **4** SERVINGS.

EASY LUNCH IDEA

LONDONER'S EGG SANDWICH

Healthy ⚥ Weight

Mix together 1 tablespoon reduced-fat cream cheese, 1 teaspoon whole-grain mustard and ½ teaspoon chopped dill. Spread the mixture over 2 toasted slices of thin whole-grain rye bread. Top one slice with a sliced hard-boiled egg, 2 slices of tomato and a pinch each of salt and pepper. Cover with the other slice of bread.

MAKES **1** SERVING.

PER SERVING: **258 CALORIES**; 10 g fat (4 g sat, 3 g mono); 220 mg cholesterol; 29 g carbohydrate; 13 g protein; 3 g fiber; 703 mg sodium; 203 mg potassium.
NUTRITION BONUS: Selenium (46% daily value), Folate (19% dv), Iron (15% dv).

GOLDEN POLENTA & EGG WITH MUSTARD SAUCE

Here's a streamlined version of Eggs Benedict: store-bought polenta, boiled eggs and an easy, no-cook homage to hollandaise. It's a quick dinner any night of the week— or a great weekend brunch.

1/2	cup low-fat plain yogurt
1/3	cup reduced-fat mayonnaise
1	tablespoon Dijon mustard
1	tablespoon lemon juice
1	tablespoon water
1	pound green beans, trimmed
4	eggs
2	teaspoons extra-virgin olive oil
1	14 ounce tube prepared polenta, sliced into eight 1/2-inch rounds

1. Combine yogurt, mayonnaise, mustard, lemon juice and water in a small bowl. Set aside.
2. Bring 6 cups of lightly salted water to a boil in a medium saucepan. Add green beans and cook until just tender, 4 minutes. Remove the green beans with a slotted spoon and divide among 4 plates.
3. Return the water to a boil; place eggs, one by one, in the boiling water and set the timer: 5 minutes for a soft-boiled egg, 8 minutes for hard-boiled. When cool enough to handle, peel and slice the eggs in half.
4. Meanwhile, heat the oil in a large nonstick skillet over medium-high heat. Add polenta rounds in a single layer and cook, turning once, until crispy and golden, about 4 minutes per side. Place 2 polenta rounds on each plate and keep warm. Add the reserved sauce to the pan and cook over medium-low heat, stirring constantly to avoid scorching, until heated through, about 3 minutes.
5. Divide the polenta rounds among the plates, top with egg halves and drizzle with the sauce. Serve immediately.

MAKES 4 SERVINGS.

PER SERVING:

287 CALORIES

13 g fat (3 g sat, 5 g mono)
219 mg cholesterol
29 g carbohydrate
13 g protein
4 g fiber
566 mg sodium
313 mg potassium

NUTRITION BONUS:
Vitamin A & Vitamin C
(20% daily value)
Calcium (15% dv)

Healthy)(Weight

ACTIVE TIME: **25 MINUTES**

TOTAL: **30 MINUTES**

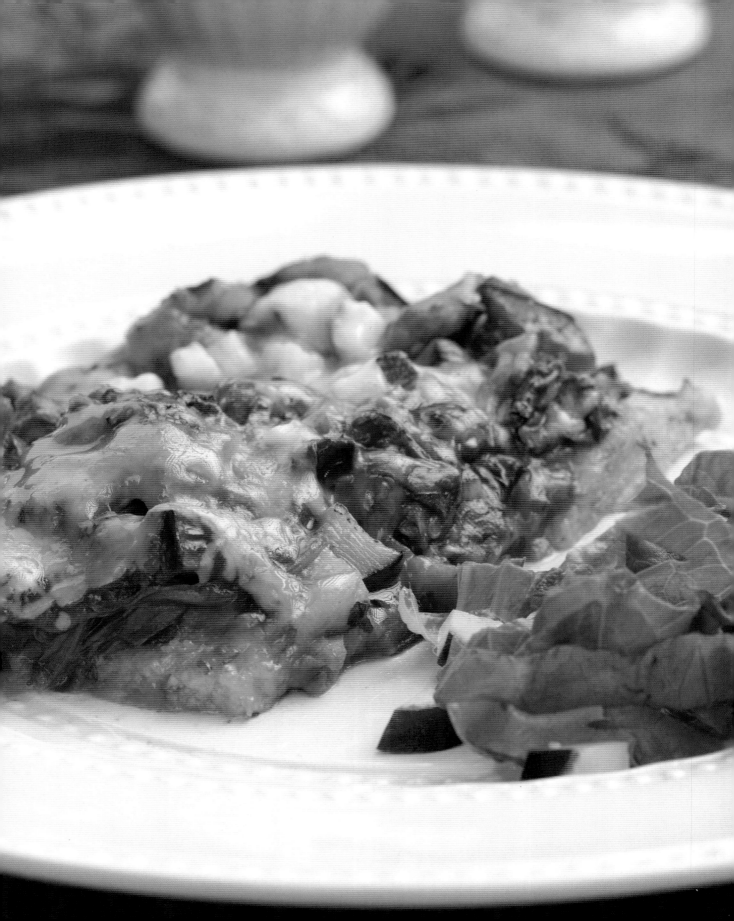

POLENTA & VEGETABLE BAKE

If you're craving eggplant parmigiana, this comforting casserole, packed with flavorful fall vegetables, fills the bill deliciously.

2	tablespoons extra-virgin olive oil
1	medium eggplant, diced
1	small zucchini, finely diced
1/2	teaspoon salt
1/2	teaspoon freshly ground pepper
1/2	cup water
1	10-ounce bag baby spinach
1 1/2	cups prepared marinara sauce, preferably lower-sodium
1/2	cup chopped fresh basil
1	14-ounce tube prepared polenta, sliced lengthwise into 6 thin slices
1 1/2	cups shredded part-skim mozzarella, divided

1. Preheat oven to 450°F. Coat a 9-by-13-inch baking dish with cooking spray.

2. Heat oil in a large nonstick skillet over medium-high heat. Add eggplant, zucchini, salt and pepper and cook, stirring occasionally, until the vegetables are tender and just beginning to brown, 4 to 6 minutes. Add water and spinach; cover and cook until wilted, stirring once, about 3 minutes. Stir marinara sauce into the vegetables and heat through, 1 to 2 minutes. Remove from the heat and stir in basil.

3. Place polenta slices in a single layer in the prepared baking dish, trimming to fit if necessary. Sprinkle with ¾ cup cheese, top with the eggplant mixture and sprinkle with the remaining ¾ cup cheese. Bake until bubbling and the cheese has just melted, 12 to 15 minutes. Let stand for about 5 minutes before serving.

MAKES 8 SERVINGS.

PER SERVING:

215 CALORIES

8 g fat (3 g sat, 4 g mono)

14 mg cholesterol

27 g carbohydrate

9 g protein

6 g fiber

670 mg sodium

187 mg potassium

NUTRITION BONUS:
Vitamin A (35% daily value)
Calcium & Vitamin C (25% dv)
Fiber (23% dv)

Healthy ⚖ Weight

High ⬆ Fiber

ACTIVE TIME: **35 MINUTES**

TOTAL: **40 MINUTES**

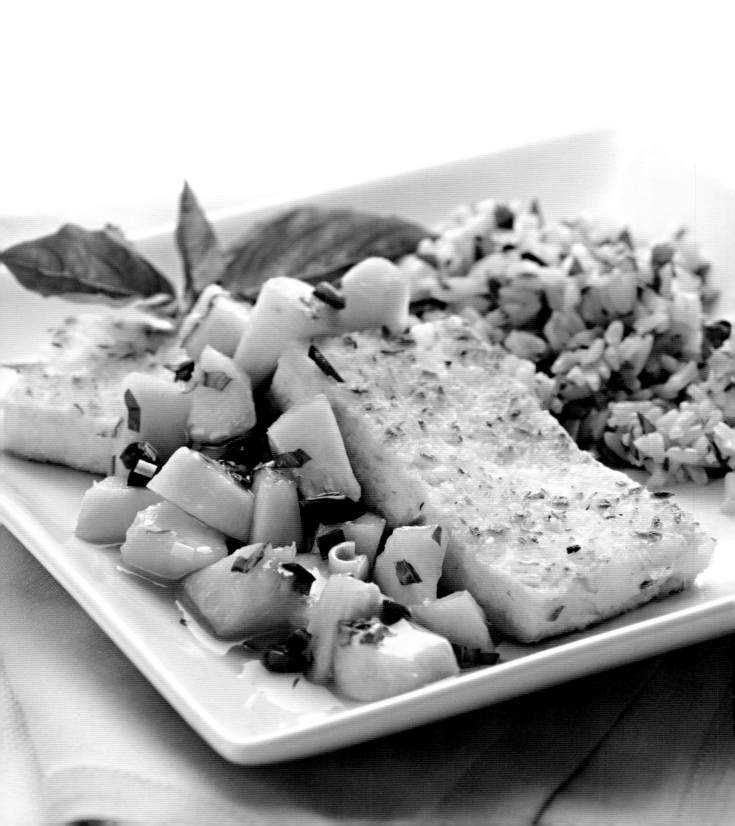

COCONUT-CRUSTED TOFU WITH PEACH-LEMONGRASS SALSA

Inspired by that restaurant-chain classic—deep-fried coconut shrimp—tofu gets an irresistibly crunchy crust and spicy-sweet salsa on the side. It's enough to convert even a confirmed tofu-phobe.

- 3 medium peaches, peeled, pitted and diced
- 1-2 jalapeños, preferably red, seeded and minced
- 1 2-inch piece fresh lemongrass, minced, *or* 1 teaspoon dried (*see Note*)
- 1 tablespoon chopped fresh basil
- 1 tablespoon brown sugar
- 1 tablespoon rice-wine vinegar
- 3/4 teaspoon salt, divided
- 1/3 cup unsweetened flaked coconut
- 2 tablespoons flour
- 2 tablespoons cornstarch
- 1 14-ounce package extra-firm water-packed tofu, drained
- 2 tablespoons canola oil, divided

1. Preheat oven to 400°F. Set a wire rack on a large baking sheet.
2. Combine peaches, jalapeños, lemongrass, basil, brown sugar, vinegar and 1/4 teaspoon salt in a medium bowl; toss to combine.
3. Mix coconut, flour and cornstarch in a shallow dish. Cut the block of tofu lengthwise into 8 thin steaks. Pat the tofu slices dry with a paper towel, sprinkle with the remaining 1/2 teaspoon salt, then press both sides of each tofu steak into the coconut mixture.
4. Heat 1 tablespoon oil in a large nonstick skillet over medium-high heat. Add 4 tofu steaks and cook until golden brown, about 2 minutes per side, adjusting heat as necessary to prevent scorching. Transfer the tofu steaks to the rack-lined baking sheet and place in the oven to keep warm. Heat the remaining 1 tablespoon oil in the skillet over medium-high heat; cook the remaining tofu steaks until golden brown, about 2 minutes per side. Serve the tofu with the peach salsa.

MAKES 4 SERVINGS, 2 TOFU STEAKS & 2/3 CUP SALSA EACH.

PER SERVING:

251 CALORIES

16 g fat (4 g sat, 9 g mono)
0 mg cholesterol
19 g carbohydrate
11 g protein
3 g fiber
491 mg sodium
313 mg potassium

NUTRITION BONUS:
Calcium (20% daily value)
Magnesium (16% dv)
Iron (15% dv)

Healthy)(Weight

Lower ⬇ Carbs

ACTIVE TIME: 35 MINUTES

TOTAL: 35 MINUTES

INGREDIENT NOTE:

- Lemongrass, essential to Thai and Vietnamese cooking, is an edible grass with bright lemon fragrance and taste. Find it fresh in the produce section of large supermarkets, at Asian food stores and chopped and dried in specialty spice sections. Purchase from Penzeys Spices, (800) 741-7787, www.penzeys.com.

221 CALORIES

14 g fat (2 g sat, 3 g mono)

0 mg cholesterol

15 g carbohydrate

12 g protein

4 g fiber

231 mg sodium

262 mg potassium

NUTRITION BONUS:
Calcium (16% daily value)
Iron (16% dv)

Healthy)(Weight

Lower ⬇ Carbs

ACTIVE TIME: **15 MINUTES**

TOTAL: **25 MINUTES**

INGREDIENT NOTE:

▪ We prefer water-packed tofu from the refrigerated section of the supermarket. Crumbling it into uneven pieces creates more surface area, improving the texture and avoiding the blocky look that turns many people away.

PEANUT-GINGER TOFU & VEGETABLES

Tofu and vegetables get a dramatic lift from a spicy peanut sauce. Serve with a cucumber salad for a low-calorie, nutrient-packed vegetarian supper.

SAUCE

5	tablespoons water
4	tablespoons smooth natural peanut butter
1	tablespoon rice vinegar (*see Ingredient Note, page 245*) *or* white vinegar
2	teaspoons reduced-sodium soy sauce
2	teaspoons honey
2	teaspoons minced ginger
2	cloves garlic, minced

TOFU & VEGETABLES

14	ounces extra-firm tofu, preferably water-packed (*see Note*)
2	teaspoons extra-virgin olive oil
4	cups baby spinach (6 ounces)
1½	cups sliced mushrooms (4 ounces)
4	scallions, sliced (1 cup)

1. TO PREPARE SAUCE: Whisk the sauce ingredients in a small bowl.

2. TO PREPARE TOFU: Drain and rinse tofu; pat dry. Slice the block crosswise into eight ½-inch-thick slabs. Coarsely crumble each slice into smaller, uneven pieces.

3. Heat oil in a large nonstick skillet over high heat. Add tofu and cook in a single layer, without stirring, until the pieces begin to turn golden brown on the bottom, about 5 minutes. Then gently stir and continue cooking, stirring occasionally, until all sides are golden brown, 5 to 7 minutes more.

4. Add spinach, mushrooms, scallions and the peanut sauce and cook, stirring, until the vegetables are just cooked, 1 to 2 minutes more.

MAKES 4 SERVINGS, GENEROUS 3/4 CUP EACH.

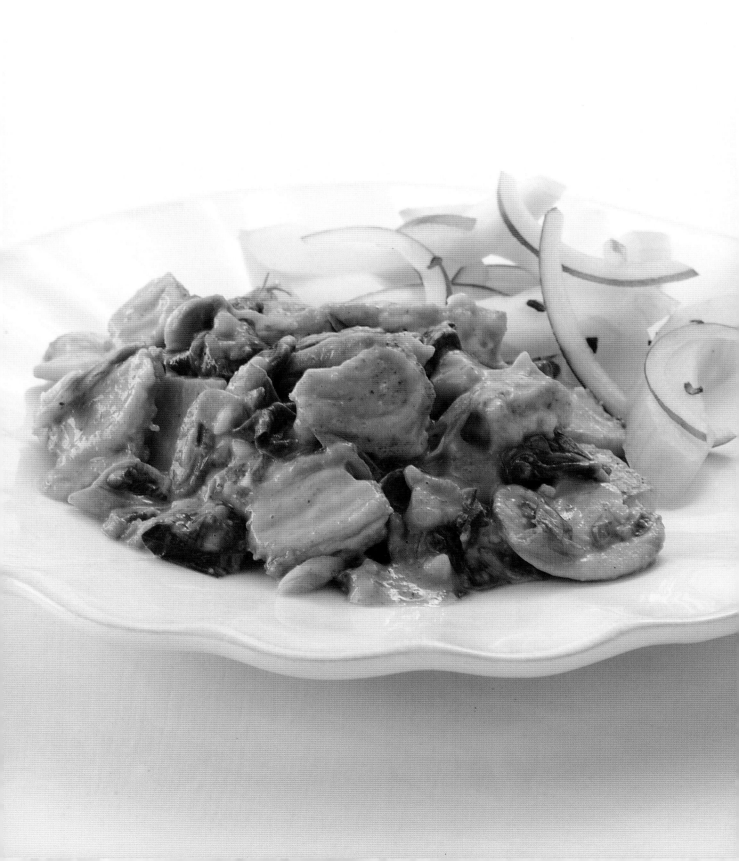

ACTIVE TIME: **20 MINUTES**

TOTAL: **20 MINUTES**

TO MAKE AHEAD: **Cover and refrigerate for up to 2 days.**

CURRIED TOFU SALAD

Call this one the EATINGWELL philosophy in a single dish: heart-healthy tofu and walnuts, ripe grapes, a few aromatics and a light version of curried mayo dressing. All together, it makes a brilliant, quick lunch or dinner.

3	tablespoons low-fat plain yogurt
2	tablespoons reduced-fat mayonnaise
2	tablespoons prepared mango chutney
2	teaspoons curry powder, preferably hot Madras
1/4	teaspoon salt
	Freshly ground pepper to taste
1	14-ounce package extra-firm water-packed tofu, drained, rinsed and finely crumbled
2	stalks celery, diced
1	cup red grapes, sliced in half
1/2	cup sliced scallions
1/4	cup chopped walnuts

Whisk yogurt, mayonnaise, chutney, curry powder, salt and pepper in a large bowl. Add tofu, celery, grapes, scallions and walnuts; stir to combine.

MAKES **6** SERVINGS, 2/3 CUP EACH.

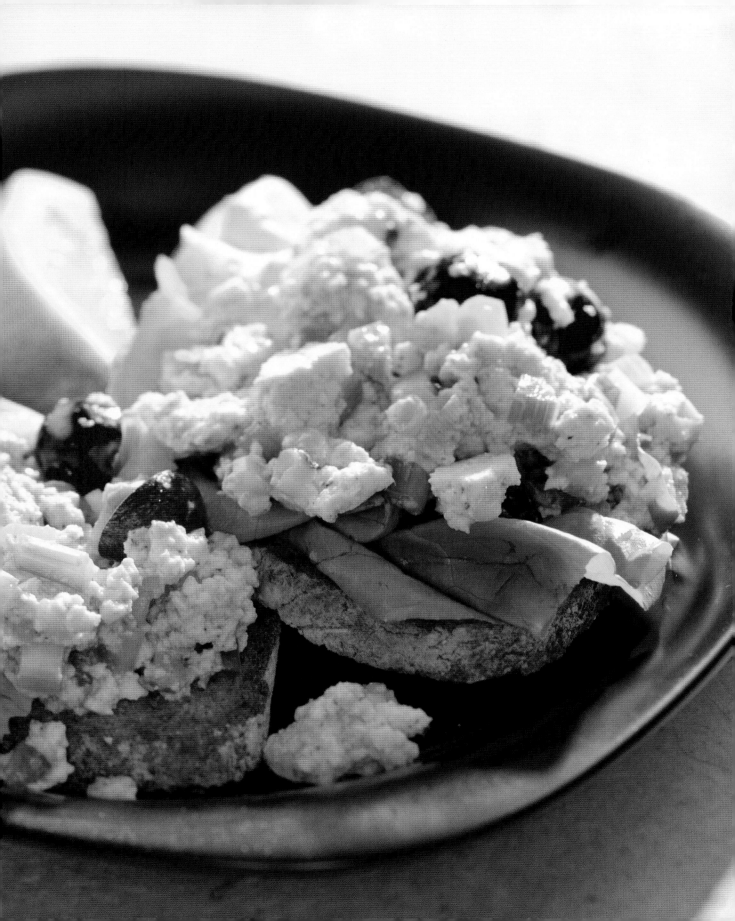

277 CALORIES

13 g fat (4 g sat, 7 g mono)

25 mg cholesterol

28 g carbohydrate

14 g protein

6 g fiber

654 mg sodium

706 mg potassium

NUTRITION BONUS:
Vitamin A (270% daily value)
Vitamin C (50% dv)
Folate (44% dv)
Calcium (35% dv)
Potassium (20% dv)

Healthy)(Weight

High ⬆ Fiber

ACTIVE TIME: **20 MINUTES**

TOTAL: **20 MINUTES**

SHOPPING TIP:

- When buying frozen ravioli or tortellini, be sure to read the label—the fat content per serving can vary widely according to brand.

FLORENTINE RAVIOLI

The flavors of Italy are best expressed in simplicity: a dash of spices, a little oil and dinner's on the table in minutes—especially if you use frozen spinach and frozen ravioli or tortellini.

1	20-ounce package frozen cheese ravioli *or* tortellini (4 cups) (*see Tip*)
6	teaspoons extra-virgin olive oil, divided
4	cloves garlic, minced
1/4	teaspoon salt
1/8-1/4	teaspoon crushed red pepper
1	16-ounce bag frozen chopped *or* whole-leaf spinach
1/2	cup water
1/4	cup freshly grated Parmesan cheese

1. Bring a large pot of water to a boil; cook ravioli (or tortellini) according to package directions.

2. Meanwhile, heat 2 teaspoons oil in a large nonstick skillet over medium heat. Add garlic and cook, stirring, until fragrant, about 30 seconds. Add salt, crushed red pepper to taste, spinach and water. Cook, stirring frequently, until the spinach has thawed, wilted and heated through, 5 to 7 minutes. Divide among 4 bowls, top with the pasta and drizzle 1 teaspoon of the remaining oil over each portion. Serve immediately with a sprinkle of Parmesan.

MAKES **4** SERVINGS, ABOUT **1 1/2** CUPS EACH.

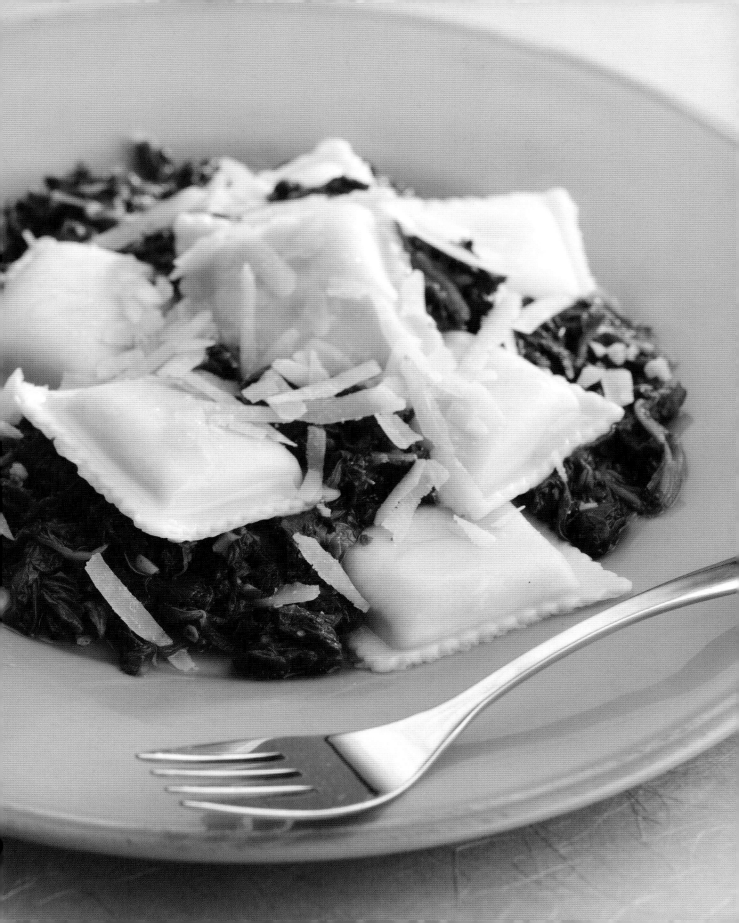

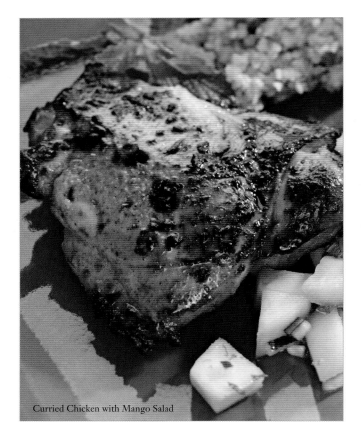

Curried Chicken with Mango Salad

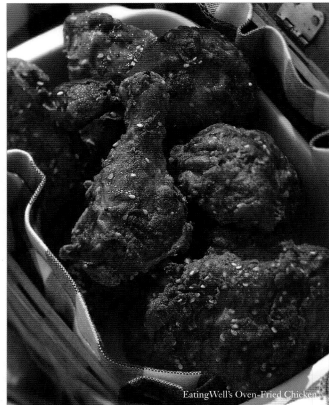

EatingWell's Oven-Fried Chicken

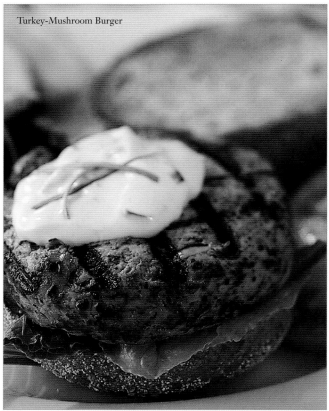

Turkey-Mushroom Burger

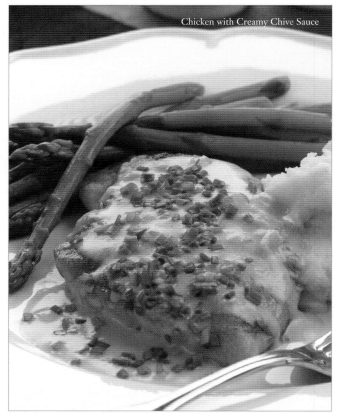

Chicken with Creamy Chive Sauce

CHICKEN & TURKEY

" Poultry is for cookery

what canvas is for painting. **"**

JEAN-ANTHELME BRILLAT-SAVARIN, CHEF, CULINARY PHILOSOPHER

ACTIVE TIME: **20 MINUTES**

TOTAL: **40 MINUTES**

INGREDIENT NOTE:

- Dried egg whites are convenient in recipes like this one because you don't have to figure out what to do with 4 leftover egg yolks. Look for powdered brands like Just Whites in the baking aisle or natural-foods section or fresh pasteurized whites in the dairy case of most supermarkets.

ALMOND-CRUSTED CHICKEN FINGERS

Instead of greasy batter, our chicken fingers are lightly coated with a spicy, crunchy ground almond and whole-wheat flour mixture. Call it fast-food for grownups, though it's still plenty kid-friendly.

	Canola oil cooking spray
½	cup sliced almonds
¼	cup whole-wheat flour
1 ½	teaspoons paprika
½	teaspoon garlic powder
½	teaspoon dry mustard
¼	teaspoon salt
⅛	teaspoon freshly ground pepper
1 ½	teaspoons extra-virgin olive oil
4	egg whites (*see Note*)
1	pound chicken tenders

1. Preheat oven to 475°F. Set a wire rack on a foil-lined baking sheet and coat with cooking spray.

2. Place almonds, flour, paprika, garlic powder, dry mustard, salt and pepper in a food processor; process until the almonds are finely chopped and the paprika is mixed throughout, about 1 minute. With the motor running, drizzle in oil; process until combined. Transfer the mixture to a shallow dish.

3. Whisk egg whites in a second shallow dish. Add chicken tenders and turn to coat. Transfer each tender to the almond mixture; turn to coat evenly. (Discard any remaining egg white and almond mixture.) Place the tenders on the prepared rack and coat with cooking spray; turn and spray the other side.

4. Bake the chicken fingers until golden brown, crispy and no longer pink in the center, 20 to 25 minutes.

MAKES **4** SERVINGS.

HAM-&-CHEESE-STUFFED CHICKEN BREASTS

Making a pocket in the chicken breast to hold the stuffing is easy with a good, sharp, thin-bladed knife. Browning the chicken in a skillet before baking gives it a beautiful golden color, and finishing in the oven ensures that it cooks evenly throughout.

- ¼ cup grated Swiss, Monterey Jack *or* part-skim mozzarella cheese
- 2 tablespoons chopped ham
- 2 teaspoons Dijon mustard
  Freshly ground pepper to taste
- 4 boneless skinless chicken breast halves (1-1 ¼ pounds total)
- 1 egg white
- ½ cup plain dry breadcrumbs
- 2 teaspoons extra-virgin olive oil

1. Preheat oven to 400°F. Use a baking sheet with sides and lightly coat it with cooking spray.
2. Mix cheese, ham, mustard and pepper in a small bowl.
3. Cut a horizontal slit along the thin, long edge of a chicken breast half, nearly through to the opposite side. Open up the breast and place one-fourth of the filling in the center. Close the breast over the filling, pressing the edges firmly together to seal. Repeat with the remaining chicken breasts and filling.
4. Lightly beat egg white with a fork in a medium bowl. Place breadcrumbs in a shallow glass dish. Hold each chicken breast half together and dip in egg white, then dredge in breadcrumbs. (Discard leftovers.)
5. Heat oil in a large nonstick skillet over medium-high heat. Add chicken breasts; cook until browned on one side, about 2 minutes. Place the chicken, browned-side up, on the prepared baking sheet. Bake until the chicken is no longer pink in the center or until an instant-read thermometer registers 170°F, about 20 minutes.

MAKES 4 SERVINGS.

PER SERVING:

236 CALORIES

7 g fat (2 g sat, 3 g mono)

74 mg cholesterol

10 g carbohydrate

31 g protein

1 g fiber

287 mg sodium

347 mg potassium

NUTRITION BONUS:
Selenium (38% daily value)

Healthy ⅓ Weight

Lower ⬇ Carbs

ACTIVE TIME: **25 MINUTES**

TOTAL: **50 MINUTES**

EATINGWELL'S OVEN-FRIED CHICKEN

Marinating the chicken legs in buttermilk keeps them juicy, and the light coating of flour, sesame seeds and spices, misted with olive oil, forms an appealing crust during baking.

½	cup buttermilk
1	tablespoon Dijon mustard
2	cloves garlic, minced
1	teaspoon hot sauce, such as Tabasco
2½-3	pounds chicken legs, skin removed, trimmed of fat
½	cup whole-wheat flour
2	tablespoons sesame seeds
1½	teaspoons paprika
1	teaspoon dried thyme
1	teaspoon baking powder
⅛	teaspoon salt
	Freshly ground pepper to taste
	Olive oil cooking spray

1. Whisk buttermilk, mustard, garlic and hot sauce in a shallow glass dish until well blended. Add chicken and turn to coat. Cover and marinate in the refrigerator for at least 30 minutes or for up to 8 hours.

2. Preheat oven to 425°F. Line a baking sheet with foil. Set a wire rack on the baking sheet and coat it with cooking spray.

3. Whisk flour, sesame seeds, paprika, thyme, baking powder, salt and pepper in a small bowl. Place the flour mixture in a paper bag or large sealable plastic bag. Shaking off excess marinade, place one or two pieces of chicken at a time in the bag and shake to coat. Shake off excess flour and place the chicken on the prepared rack. (Discard any leftover flour mixture and marinade.) Spray the chicken pieces with cooking spray.

4. Bake the chicken until golden brown and no longer pink in the center, 40 to 50 minutes.

MAKES **4** SERVINGS.

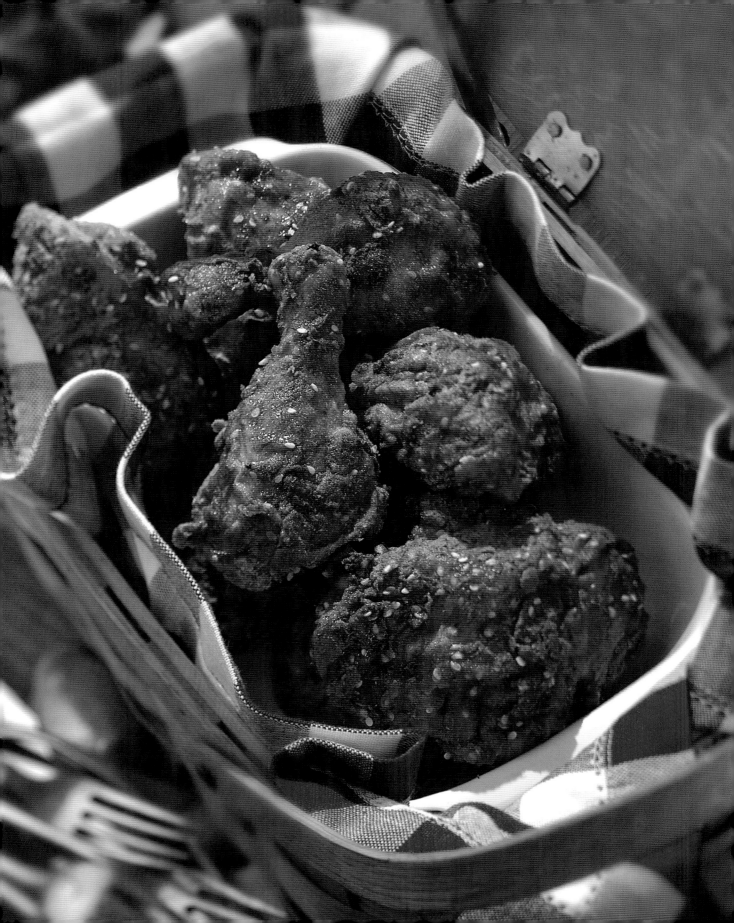

312 CALORIES

11 g fat (4 g sat, 4 g mono)

76 mg cholesterol

19 g carbohydrate

35 g protein

4 g fiber

652 mg sodium

402 mg potassium

NUTRITION BONUS:
Vitamin C (70% daily value)
Vitamin A (35% dv)
Calcium (30% dv)
Folate (19% dv)

Healthy)(Weight

Lower ⬇ Carbs

ACTIVE TIME: **30 MINUTES**

TOTAL: **1 HOUR**

TO CLEAN LEEKS:

■ Trim roots and ragged tops. Slice leeks and place in plenty of water, then drain. Repeat a few times. The slices do not absorb water or lose flavor.

CHICKEN DIVAN

This '50s-era staple, proudly made with canned soup and frozen broccoli, never went out of style. We've given it a healthier update without losing its comfort-food appeal. Use leftover cooked chicken breasts, if you have them on hand, for an even faster dinner.

1 ½   pounds boneless, skinless chicken breast
1   tablespoon extra-virgin olive oil
2   cups diced leek, white and light green parts only (about 1 large; *see Tip*)
½   teaspoon salt
5   tablespoons all-purpose flour
1   14-ounce can reduced-sodium chicken broth
1   cup 1% milk
2   tablespoons dry sherry (*see Note, page 245*)
½   teaspoon dried thyme
½   teaspoon freshly ground pepper
2   10-ounce boxes frozen chopped broccoli, thawed, *or* 1 pound broccoli crowns, chopped
1   cup grated Parmesan cheese, divided
¼   cup reduced-fat mayonnaise
2   teaspoons Dijon mustard

1. Preheat oven to 375°F. Coat a 7-by-11-inch (2 quart) glass baking dish with cooking spray.
2. Place chicken in a medium skillet or saucepan and add lightly salted water to cover. Bring to a simmer over high heat. Cover, reduce heat to low and simmer gently until the chicken is cooked through and no longer pink in the center, 10 to 12 minutes. Drain and slice into bite-size pieces.
3. Heat oil in a large nonstick skillet over medium-high heat. Add leek and salt and cook, stirring often, until softened but not browned, 3 to 4 minutes. Add flour; stir to coat. Add broth, milk, sherry, thyme and pepper and bring to a simmer, stirring constantly. Add broccoli; return to a simmer. Remove from heat and stir in ½ cup Parmesan, mayonnaise and mustard.
4. Spread half the broccoli mixture in the prepared baking dish. Top with the chicken, then the remaining broccoli mixture. Sprinkle evenly with the remaining ½ cup Parmesan. Bake until bubbling, 20 to 25 minutes. Let cool for 10 minutes before serving.

MAKES **6** SERVINGS, ABOUT **1** ⅓ CUPS EACH.

SPICY CHICKEN TACOS

While many North Americans think of tacos as having crisp, fried shells, authentic Mexican tacos are made with soft, fresh corn tortillas. The traditional preparation is the smart choice, as unfried corn tortillas are low in fat and made with whole grains.

- 8 corn tortillas
- 1 pound boneless, skinless chicken breasts, trimmed of fat and cut into thin strips
- ¼ teaspoon salt, or to taste
- 2 teaspoons canola oil, divided
- 1 large onion, sliced
- 1 large green bell pepper, seeded and sliced
- 3 large cloves garlic, minced
- 1 jalapeño pepper, seeded and minced
- 1 tablespoon ground cumin
- ½ cup prepared hot salsa, plus more for garnish
- ¼ cup chopped fresh cilantro
  Sliced scallions, chopped fresh tomatoes and reduced-fat sour cream for garnish

1. Preheat oven to 300°F. Wrap tortillas in foil and bake until heated through, 10 to 15 minutes.
2. Meanwhile, season chicken with salt. Heat 1 teaspoon oil in a large heavy skillet over high heat until very hot. Add chicken and cook, stirring until browned on all sides, about 6 minutes. Transfer to a bowl.
3. Reduce heat to medium and add the remaining 1 teaspoon oil to skillet. Add onion and cook, stirring, until they start to brown around the edges, 3 to 5 minutes. Add bell pepper, garlic, jalapeño and cumin. Cook, stirring, until peppers are bright green but still crisp, 2 to 3 minutes more.
4. Stir in salsa and reserved chicken. Cook, stirring, until chicken is heated through, about 2 minutes. Remove from heat and stir in cilantro. Spoon into warmed tortillas and garnish with scallions, tomatoes and sour cream.

MAKES 4 SERVINGS, 2 TACOS EACH.

PER SERVING (WITHOUT GARNISHES):

303 CALORIES

6 g fat (1 g sat, 2 g mono)
66 mg cholesterol
32 g carbohydrate
31 g protein
5 g fiber
420 mg sodium
533 mg potassium

NUTRITION BONUS:
Vitamin C (68% daily value)
Folate (25% dv)
Fiber (20% dv)

Healthy)(Weight

High ↑ Fiber

ACTIVE TIME: **20 MINUTES**

TOTAL: **35 MINUTES**

PER SERVING:

224 CALORIES

5 g fat (1 g sat, 2 g mono)

48 mg cholesterol

26 g carbohydrate

26 g protein

8 g fiber

692 mg sodium

439 mg potassium

NUTRITION BONUS:
Fiber (31% daily value)
Folate (30% dv)

Healthy)(Weight

High ⬆ Fiber

ACTIVE TIME: **35 MINUTES**

TOTAL: **35 MINUTES**

GOLDEN CHICKEN WITH SPICY REFRIED BEANS

Kids love this combination of refried white beans and chicken tenders. If you're concerned about making it too spicy, omit the jalapeño. Serve with extra cheese to sprinkle on top.

2	teaspoons ground cumin
2	teaspoons ground coriander
¼	teaspoon freshly ground pepper
¼	teaspoon kosher salt
1	pound chicken tenders
3	teaspoons canola oil, divided
1	small onion, chopped
1	jalapeño pepper, chopped
2	15-ounce cans white beans, rinsed
¾	cup canned diced tomatoes with green chiles *or* tomato salsa
¼	cup shredded Monterey Jack *or* Cheddar cheese

1. Combine cumin, coriander, pepper and salt in a medium bowl. Add chicken and toss to coat.

2. Heat 2 teaspoons oil in a large nonstick skillet over medium-high heat. Add the chicken and sauté until golden brown and just cooked through, 2 to 4 minutes per side. Transfer to a plate and cover to keep warm.

3. Reduce heat to medium and add the remaining 1 teaspoon oil to the pan. Add onion and jalapeño and cook until beginning to soften, 1 to 2 minutes. Add beans, tomatoes (or salsa) and any accumulated juices from the chicken; cook, stirring often, until heated through, about 3 minutes. Transfer the bean mixture to a medium bowl and mash with a potato masher until creamy but still slightly chunky. Stir in cheese. Serve with the chicken.

MAKES **6** SERVINGS.

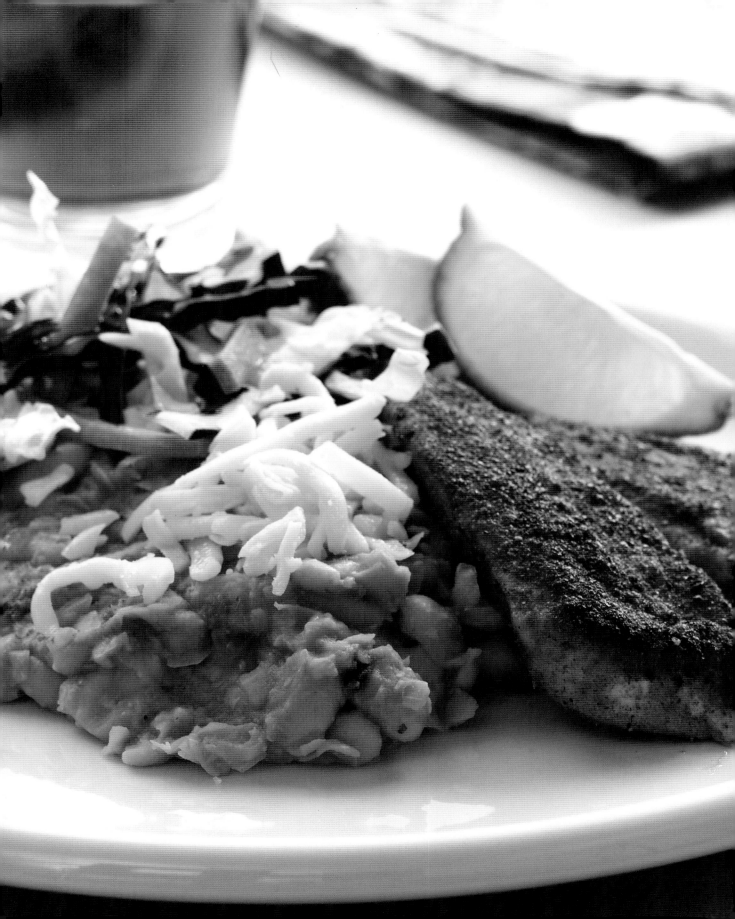

ACTIVE TIME: **35 MINUTES**

TOTAL: **2 HOURS**

TEMPERATURE CHECK

- The best way to determine if poultry is fully cooked is to use an instant-read thermometer. The internal temperature should register 165°F for a whole chicken. (To check, insert the thermometer into the thickest part of the thigh.)

HERB & LEMON ROAST CHICKEN

Even if you're only feeding four, it is a good idea to roast two chickens at once. It takes the same amount of time and then you have leftovers to use for sandwiches, soup or salad.

2	lemons
2	cups packed parsley leaves
¼	cup fresh thyme leaves
¼	cup fresh rosemary leaves
3	cloves garlic, peeled
1½	tablespoons extra-virgin olive oil
2	teaspoons salt
	Freshly ground pepper to taste
2	whole chickens (3½-4 pounds each)
1	14½-ounce can reduced-sodium chicken broth, divided
½	cup dry white wine
2	tablespoons water mixed with 1 tablespoon cornstarch

1. Position oven rack in lower third of oven; preheat to 350°F. Coat a large roasting pan with cooking spray.

2. TO PREPARE CHICKENS: Zest lemons, then cut in half. Combine lemon zest, parsley, thyme, rosemary, garlic, oil, salt and pepper in a food processor or blender; process until finely chopped. Reserve ¼ cup of the mixture, covered, in the refrigerator for the gravy.

3. Place chicken hearts, necks and gizzards in the prepared pan (reserve livers for another use). Remove excess fat from chickens. Dry insides with a paper towel. With your fingers, loosen skin over breasts and thighs to make pockets, being careful not to tear the skin.

4. Spread ¼ cup herb mixture in the pan; place the chickens on top, at least 1 inch apart. Rub 1 tablespoon herb mixture into each cavity; spread remaining mixture under skin. Place 2 lemon halves in each cavity. Tuck wings behind the back and tie legs together.

5. Roast the chickens for 20 minutes. Drizzle with ¼ cup chicken broth and roast for 40 minutes more, basting with pan drippings every 20 minutes. Tent with foil and continue roasting until cooked through (*see Tip*) and juices run clear, about 30 minutes.

6. TO PREPARE GRAVY: Transfer the chickens to a platter; tent with foil. Pour pan juices into a bowl, leaving giblets in the pan. Chill juices in the freezer for 10 minutes. Meanwhile, add wine and remaining broth to the pan; bring to a boil over medium heat, scraping up any browned bits. Add any juices accumulated on the platter.

7. Skim fat from the chilled juices. Add juices to the pan; return to a boil, then strain into a saucepan. Bring to a simmer. Whisk in cornstarch mixture. Simmer, stirring, until slightly thickened, about 1 minute. Stir in reserved herb mixture. Season with pepper.

8. Carve the chickens, discarding skin. Serve with the gravy.

MAKES 8 SERVINGS.

CREAMY TARRAGON CHICKEN SALAD

Heart-healthy grapes and walnuts, crisp celery, and a simple, creamy dressing make this chicken salad elegant enough for company. Serve it on a bed of salad greens or make an open-faced sandwich on toasted whole-wheat bread slices.

2	pounds boneless, skinless chicken breasts, trimmed of fat
1	cup reduced-sodium chicken broth
1/3	cup walnuts, chopped
2/3	cup reduced-fat sour cream
1/2	cup reduced-fat mayonnaise
1	tablespoon dried tarragon
1/2	teaspoon salt
1/2	teaspoon freshly ground pepper
1 1/2	cups diced celery
1 1/2	cups halved red seedless grapes

1. Preheat oven to 450°F.

2. Arrange chicken in a glass baking dish large enough to hold it in a single layer. Pour broth around the chicken. Bake the chicken until no longer pink in the center and an instant-read thermometer inserted in the thickest part of the breast registers 170°F, 30 to 35 minutes. Transfer the chicken to a cutting board until cool enough to handle, then cut into cubes. (Discard broth or save for another use.)

3. Meanwhile, spread walnuts on a baking sheet and toast in the oven until lightly golden and fragrant, about 6 minutes. Let cool.

4. Stir sour cream, mayonnaise, tarragon, salt and pepper together in a large bowl. Add celery, grapes, the chicken and walnuts; stir to coat. Refrigerate until chilled, at least 1 hour.

MAKES 8 SERVINGS, 1 CUP EACH.

PER SERVING:

227 CALORIES

10 g fat (3 g sat, 2 g mono)

70 mg cholesterol

10 g carbohydrate

25 g protein

1 g fiber

357 mg sodium

368 mg potassium

NUTRITION BONUS:
Selenium (30% daily value)

Healthy)(Weight

Lower ⬇ Carbs

ACTIVE TIME: **30 MINUTES**

TOTAL: **1 3/4 HOURS**

TO MAKE AHEAD: **Bake the chicken (Steps 1-2) and refrigerate for up to 2 days. Cover and refrigerate the salad for up to 1 day; add the nuts just before serving.**

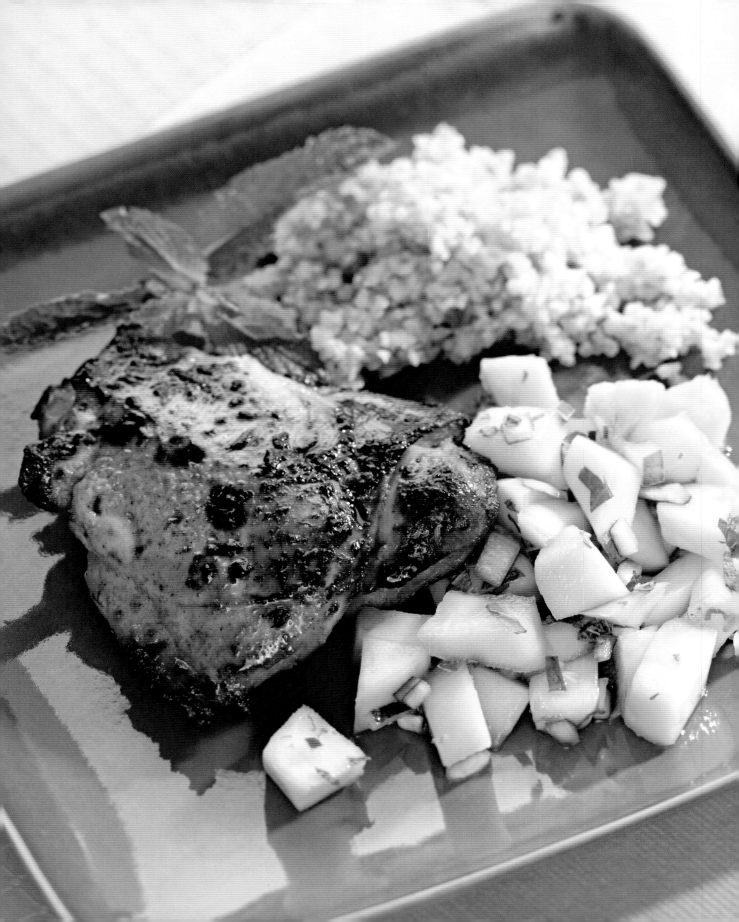

CURRIED CHICKEN WITH MANGO SALAD

If you have the time, marinate the chicken in the tangy yogurt sauce at least an hour ahead in the refrigerator, to make it even more tender and delectably juicy. You can cook the chicken on the grill if you prefer; grill on high heat, 6 to 8 minutes per side.

- ½   cup low-fat plain yogurt
- 2   tablespoons mango chutney
- 2   teaspoons garam masala (*see Note*) *or* curry powder, mild *or* hot
- 4   bone-in chicken thighs (1 ¾-2 pounds), skin removed, trimmed of fat
- ½   teaspoon kosher salt, divided
- 1   mango, diced
- ¼   cup finely diced red onion
- 2   tablespoons finely chopped fresh mint
- 2   tablespoons red-wine vinegar
- 2   teaspoons brown sugar

1. Position rack in upper third of oven; preheat broiler. Coat a broiler pan with cooking spray.
2. Whisk yogurt, chutney and garam masala (or curry powder) in a medium bowl. Add chicken; turn to coat. Remove the chicken from the sauce and transfer to the prepared broiler pan; sprinkle with ¼ teaspoon salt.
3. Broil the chicken until the coating is charred in spots, 12 to 15 minutes. Turn the chicken over and continue cooking until it is slightly charred and cooked through, 12 to 15 minutes more.
4. Meanwhile, combine mango, onion, mint, vinegar, brown sugar and the remaining ¼ teaspoon salt in a medium bowl. Serve the chicken with the mango salad.

MAKES 4 SERVINGS, 1 THIGH & ABOUT ½ CUP SALAD EACH.

PER SERVING:

289 CALORIES

12 g fat (3 g sat, 5 g mono)
101 mg cholesterol
16 g carbohydrate
29 g protein
1 g fiber
308 mg sodium
403 mg potassium

NUTRITION BONUS:
Selenium (46% daily value)
Vitamin C (25% dv)
Zinc (20% dv)

Healthy)(Weight

Lower ⬇ Carbs

ACTIVE TIME: **30 MINUTES**

TOTAL: **45 MINUTES**

INGREDIENT NOTE:

- Garam masala is a fragrant blend of ground spices commonly used in Indian cooking. It's in the spice section of most supermarkets and specialty stores.

213 CALORIES

8 g fat (1 g sat, 5 g mono)

68 mg cholesterol

10 g carbohydrate

27 g protein

0 g fiber

246 mg sodium

55 mg potassium

Healthy ⅓ Weight

Lower 🔽 Carbs

ACTIVE TIME: **20 MINUTES**

TOTAL: **20 MINUTES**

MARMALADE CHICKEN

Don't be fooled by the title: the deliciously tangy sauce in this simple chicken dish has only a hint of sweetness. Serve it with brown rice to soak up the sauce.

1	cup reduced-sodium chicken broth
2	tablespoons red-wine vinegar
2	tablespoons orange marmalade
1	teaspoon Dijon mustard
1	teaspoon cornstarch
1	pound chicken tenders
1/2	teaspoon kosher salt
1/4	teaspoon freshly ground pepper
6	teaspoons extra-virgin olive oil, divided
2	large shallots, minced
1	teaspoon freshly grated orange zest

1. Whisk broth, vinegar, marmalade, mustard and cornstarch in a medium bowl.

2. Sprinkle chicken with salt and pepper. Heat 4 teaspoons oil in a large skillet over medium-high heat. Add the chicken and cook until golden, about 2 minutes per side. Transfer to a plate and cover with foil to keep warm.

3. Add the remaining 2 teaspoons oil and shallots to the pan and cook, stirring often, until the shallots begin to brown, about 30 seconds. Whisk the broth mixture and add it to the pan. Bring to a simmer, scraping up any browned bits with a wooden spoon. Reduce heat to maintain a simmer; cook until the sauce is slightly reduced, 30 seconds to 1 minute. Add the chicken; return to a simmer. Cook, turning once, until the chicken is heated through, about 1 minute. Remove from the heat and stir in orange zest.

MAKES **4** SERVINGS.

CHICKEN WITH CREAMY CHIVE SAUCE

You'll love this ultra-creamy sauce with chicken, but it's equally wonderful with pork cutlets. Try it with cauliflower or asparagus, steamed tender-crisp, and some crusty whole-grain bread.

4	boneless, skinless chicken breasts (about 1 pound), trimmed of fat
1	teaspoon kosher salt, divided
1/4	cup plus 1 tablespoon all-purpose flour, divided
3	teaspoons extra-virgin olive oil, divided
2	large shallots, finely chopped
1/2	cup dry white wine
1	14-ounce can reduced-sodium chicken broth
1/3	cup reduced-fat sour cream
1	tablespoon Dijon mustard
1/2	cup chopped chives (about 1 bunch)

1. Place chicken between sheets of plastic wrap and pound with a meat mallet or heavy skillet until flattened to an even thickness, about 1/2 inch. Season both sides of the chicken with 1/2 teaspoon salt. Place 1/4 cup flour in a shallow glass baking dish and dredge the chicken in it. Discard the remaining flour.

2. Heat 2 teaspoons oil in a large nonstick skillet over medium-high heat. Add the chicken and cook until golden brown, 1 to 2 minutes per side. Transfer to a plate, cover and keep warm.

3. Heat the remaining 1 teaspoon oil in the pan over medium-high heat. Add shallots and cook, stirring constantly and scraping up any browned bits, until golden brown, 1 to 2 minutes. Sprinkle with the remaining 1 tablespoon flour; stir to coat. Add wine, broth and the remaining 1/2 teaspoon salt; bring to a boil, stirring often. Return the chicken and any accumulated juices to the pan, reduce heat to a simmer, and cook until heated through and no longer pink in the center, about 6 minutes. Stir in sour cream and mustard until smooth; turn the chicken to coat with the sauce. Stir in chives and serve immediately.

MAKES 4 SERVINGS.

PER SERVING:

248 CALORIES

9 g fat (3 g sat, 4 g mono)

72 mg cholesterol

9 g carbohydrate

26 g protein

0 g fiber

488 mg sodium

331 mg potassium

NUTRITION BONUS:
Niacin (50% daily value)
Selenium (31% dv)

Healthy ⧗ Weight

Lower ⬇ Carbs

ACTIVE TIME: **35 MINUTES**

TOTAL: **35 MINUTES**

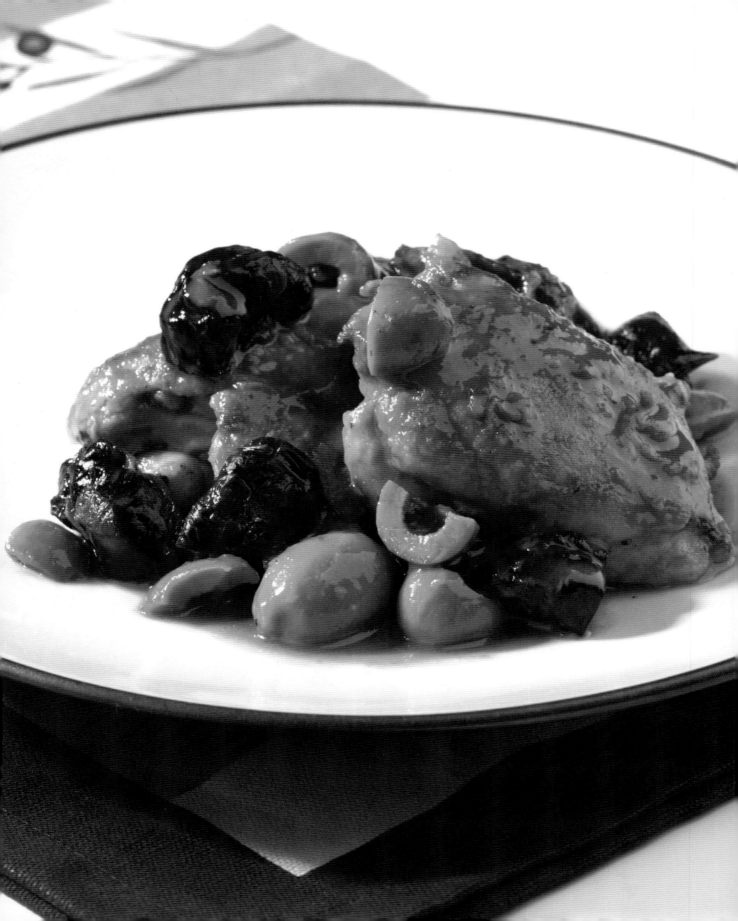

CHICKEN WITH GREEN OLIVES & PRUNES

The delicious combination of sweet, tart and savory flavors makes this simple dish the star of a weeknight meal. Serve with whole-wheat couscous, to soak up the tasty sauce, and Trio of Peas (page 224).

1 1/4	pounds boneless, skinless chicken thighs, trimmed
1	teaspoon extra-virgin olive oil
1	cup reduced-sodium chicken broth
1/4	cup red-wine vinegar
1/4	cup chopped pitted green olives, such as Spanish, Cerignola *or* cracked green
1/4	cup chopped pitted prunes (dried plums)
	Freshly ground pepper to taste

Pat chicken dry with a paper towel. Heat oil in a large nonstick skillet over medium-high heat. Add the chicken and cook until browned, about 2 minutes per side. Add broth and vinegar to the pan; bring to a simmer, stirring. Add olives, prunes and pepper; reduce heat to low. Cover and cook until the chicken is tender and no longer pink in the center, 12 to 15 minutes. Transfer the chicken to a plate. Spoon sauce over the chicken and serve.

MAKES 4 SERVINGS.

PER SERVING:

224 CALORIES

8 g fat (2 g sat, 4 g mono)

118 mg cholesterol

7 g carbohydrate

29 g protein

1 g fiber

394 mg sodium

454 mg potassium

NUTRITION BONUS:
Selenium (27% daily value)
Zinc (18% dv)

Healthy)(Weight

Lower ⬇ Carbs

ACTIVE TIME: **10 MINUTES**

TOTAL: **30 MINUTES**

ACTIVE TIME: **30 MINUTES**

TOTAL: **30 MINUTES**

TO MAKE AHEAD: **Add everything except the blueberries and dressing to the pasta salad. Cover and refrigerate pasta salad, blueberries and dressing separately for up to 1 day. Toss together just before serving.**

CHICKEN & BLUEBERRY PASTA SALAD

Wake up your palate with a surprising (and healthful) combination that works beautifully. The addition of poached chicken and feta cheese makes this dish into a light and satisfying summer supper that's also great for a potluck. If you already have some leftover chicken, skip Step 1 and add shredded chicken in Step 4.

1 pound boneless, skinless chicken breast, trimmed of fat
8 ounces whole-wheat fusilli *or* radiatore
3 tablespoons extra-virgin olive oil
1 large shallot, thinly sliced
1/3 cup reduced-sodium chicken broth
1/3 cup crumbled feta cheese
3 tablespoons lime juice
1 cup fresh blueberries
1 tablespoon chopped fresh thyme
1 teaspoon freshly grated lime zest
1/4 teaspoon salt

1. Place chicken in a skillet or saucepan and add enough water to cover; bring to a boil. Cover, reduce heat to low and simmer gently until cooked through and no longer pink in the middle, 10 to 12 minutes. Transfer the chicken to a cutting board to cool. Shred into bite-size strips.
2. Bring a large pot of water to a boil. Cook pasta until just tender, about 9 minutes or according to package directions. Drain. Place in a large bowl.
3. Meanwhile, place oil and shallot in a small skillet and cook over medium-low heat, stirring occasionally, until softened and just beginning to brown, 2 to 5 minutes. Add broth, feta and lime juice and cook, stirring occasionally, until the feta begins to melt, 1 to 2 minutes.
4. Add the chicken to the bowl with the pasta. Add the dressing, blueberries, thyme, lime zest and salt and toss until combined.

MAKES **6** SERVINGS, ABOUT 1 1/2 CUPS EACH.

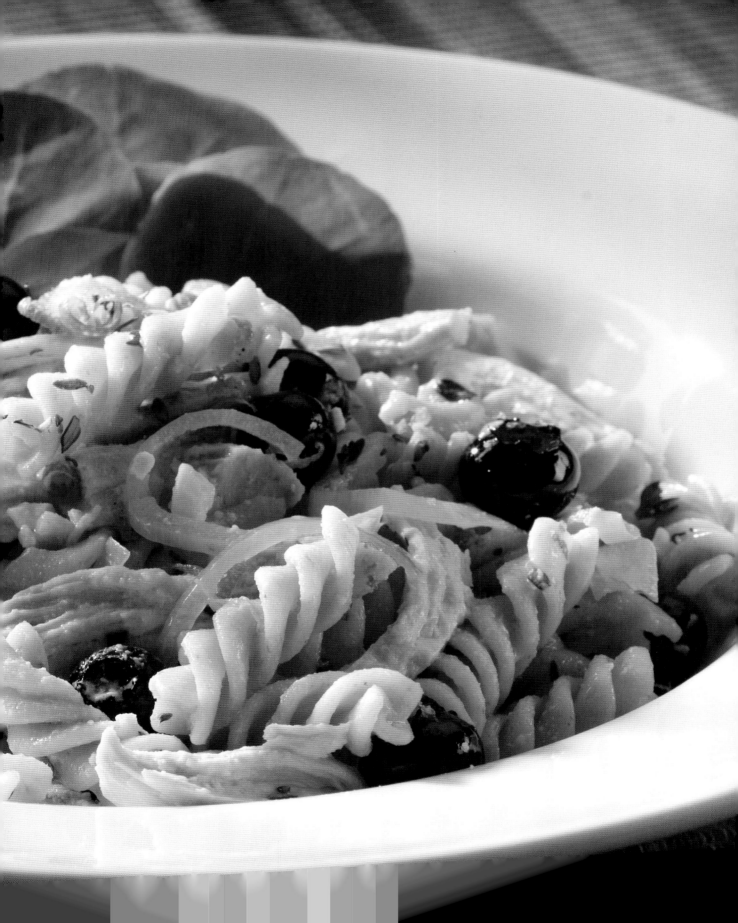

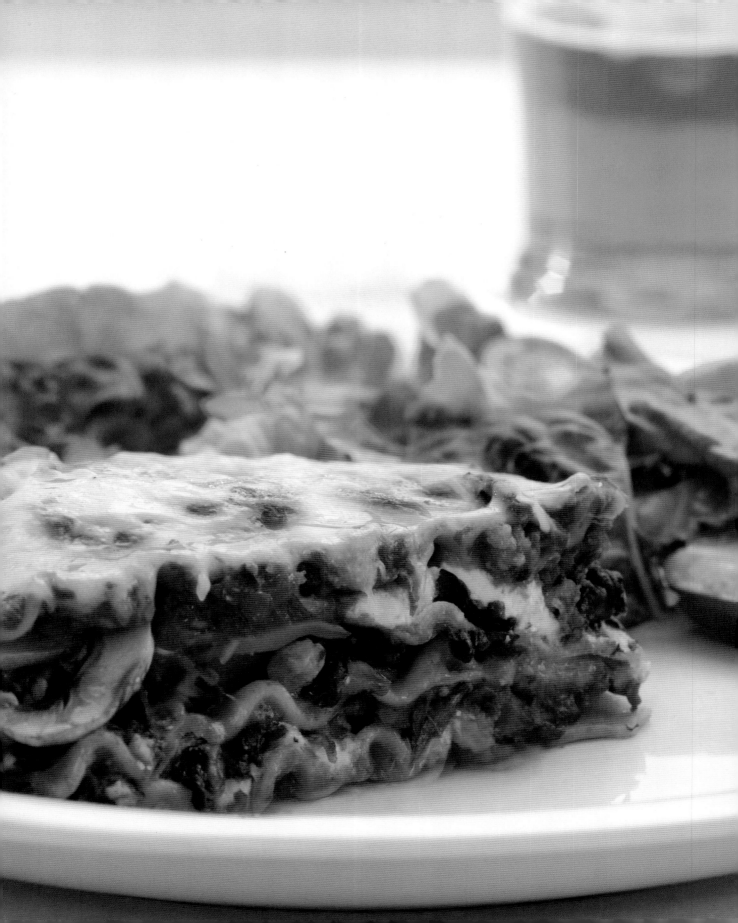

MUSHROOM, SAUSAGE & SPINACH LASAGNA

This hearty lasagna is packed with vegetables, and gets a little kick from spicy (or "hot") turkey sausage. When buying the sausage, choose the one with the lowest fat and sodium, since brands can vary widely.

8	ounces lasagna noodles, preferably whole-wheat
1	pound lean spicy Italian turkey sausage, casings removed (*see Variation*)
4	cups sliced mushrooms (10 ounces)
1/4	cup water
1	pound frozen spinach, thawed
1	28-ounce can crushed tomatoes, preferably chunky
1/4	cup chopped fresh basil
	Salt & freshly ground pepper to taste
1	pound part-skim ricotta cheese (2 cups)
8	ounces part-skim mozzarella cheese, shredded (about 2 cups), divided

1. Preheat oven to 350°F. Coat a 9-by-13-inch glass baking dish with cooking spray. Put a large pot of water on to boil.

2. Cook noodles in the boiling water until not quite al dente, about 2 minutes less than the package directions. Drain; return the noodles to the pot, cover with cool water and set aside.

3. Coat a large nonstick skillet with cooking spray and heat over medium-high heat. Add sausage and cook, crumbling with a wooden spoon, until browned, about 4 minutes. Add mushrooms and water; cook, stirring occasionally and crumbling the sausage more, until the sausage is cooked through, the water has evaporated and the mushrooms are tender, 8 to 10 minutes. Squeeze spinach to remove excess water, then stir into the pan; remove from heat.

4. Mix tomatoes with basil, salt and pepper in a medium bowl.

5. TO ASSEMBLE LASAGNA: Spread 1/2 cup of the tomatoes in the prepared baking dish. Arrange a layer of noodles on top, trimming to fit if necessary. Evenly dollop half the ricotta over the noodles. Top with half the sausage mixture, one-third of the remaining tomatoes and one-third of the mozzarella. Continue with another layer of noodles, the remaining ricotta, the remaining sausage, half the remaining tomatoes and half the remaining mozzarella. Top with a third layer of noodles and the remaining tomatoes.

6. Cover the lasagna with foil and bake until bubbling and heated through, 1 hour to 1 hour 10 minutes. Remove the foil; sprinkle the remaining mozzarella on top. Return to the oven and bake until the cheese is just melted but not browned, 8 to 10 minutes. Let rest for 10 minutes before serving.

MAKES **10** SERVINGS.

PER SERVING:

327 CALORIES

14 g fat (5 g sat, 3 g mono)
41 mg cholesterol
27 g carbohydrate
25 g protein
6 g fiber
582 mg sodium
562 mg potassium

NUTRITION BONUS:
Vitamin A (90% daily value)
Calcium (35% dv)
Folate (15% dv)

Healthy ⌇ Weight

High ⬆ Fiber

ACTIVE TIME: **30 MINUTES**

TOTAL: **2 HOURS**

TO MAKE AHEAD: **Prepare through Step 5 up to 1 day ahead.**

VEGETARIAN VARIATION:

▪ Use a sausage-style soy product, such as Gimme Lean, or simply omit the sausage altogether.

193 CALORIES

10 g fat (2 g sat, 5 g mono)

95 mg cholesterol

9 g carbohydrate

17 g protein

2 g fiber

419 mg sodium

385 mg potassium

NUTRITION BONUS:
Potassium (19% daily value)

Healthy ⊃⊂ Weight

Lower ⬇ Carbs

ACTIVE TIME: **45 MINUTES**

TOTAL: **1 HOUR**

TO MAKE AHEAD: **Prepare
patties through Step 4. Wrap
individually and refrigerate
for up to 8 hours or freeze
for up to 3 months. Thaw in
the refrigerator before
cooking.**

INGREDIENT NOTE:

▪ Check labels carefully and
select ground turkey breast.
Regular ground turkey,
which is a mixture of dark
and white meat, has a
higher fat content (similar
to that of lean ground beef).

TURKEY-MUSHROOM BURGERS

*Ground turkey is the standard lean alternative to ground beef, but burgers
made from it can be dry, bland and—well, a little pale-looking. We've solved those
problems by extending the ground meat with mushrooms, producing an uncom-
monly juicy, flavorful burger.*

2	slices whole-wheat sandwich bread, crusts removed, torn into pieces
8	ounces white mushrooms, wiped clean
3	teaspoons extra-virgin olive oil, divided
1	medium onion, finely chopped
2	cloves garlic, minced
1	pound lean ground turkey breast (*see Note*)
1	large egg, lightly beaten
3	tablespoons chopped fresh dill
1 ½	tablespoons coarse-grained mustard
½	teaspoon salt
¼	teaspoon freshly ground pepper
6	whole-wheat buns (optional)
	Lettuce leaves & tomato slices for garnish

1. Place bread in a food processor and pulse into fine crumbs. Transfer to a
large bowl. Pulse mushrooms in the food processor until finely chopped.

2. Heat 2 teaspoons oil in a large nonstick skillet over medium-high heat.
Add the onion, garlic and mushrooms; cook, stirring occasionally, until
tender and liquid has evaporated, about 10 minutes. Add to breadcrumbs
and let cool completely, 15 to 20 minutes.

3. Preheat grill to medium-high.

4. Add ground turkey, egg, dill, mustard, salt and pepper to the mushroom
mixture; mix well with a potato masher. With dampened hands, form the
mixture into six ½-inch-thick patties, using about ⅛ cup for each.

5. Oil the grill rack (*see Tip, page 245*). Brush the patties with the remaining
1 teaspoon oil. Grill until no longer pink in the center, about 5 minutes per
side. (An instant-read thermometer inserted in the center should register
165°F.) Meanwhile, split buns and toast on the grill for 30 to 60 seconds, if
using. Serve burgers on buns, garnished with lettuce and tomato, if desired.

MAKES **6** SERVINGS.

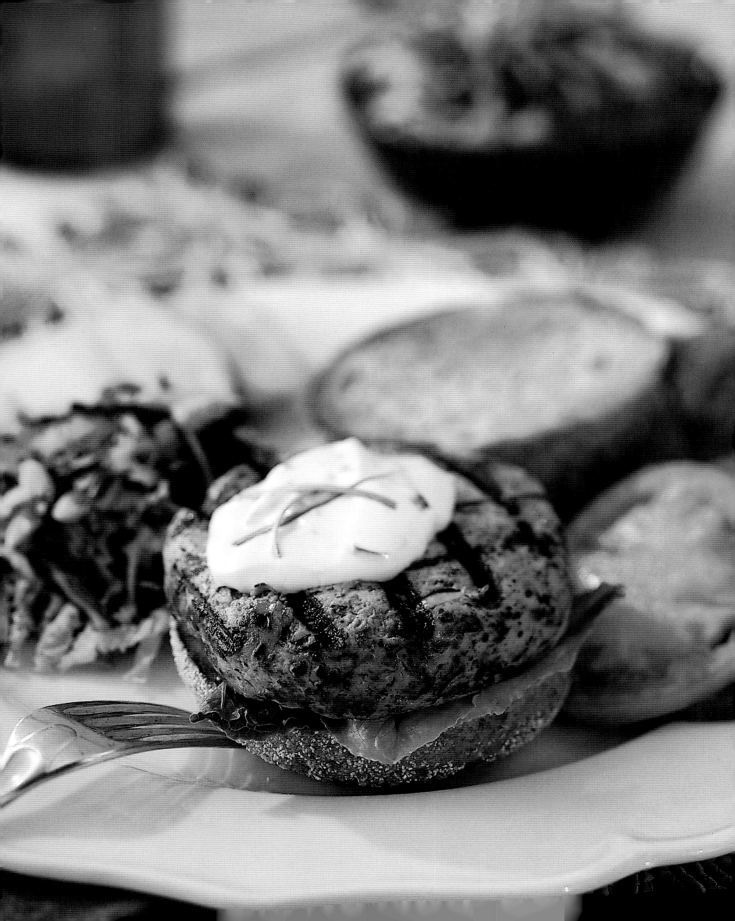

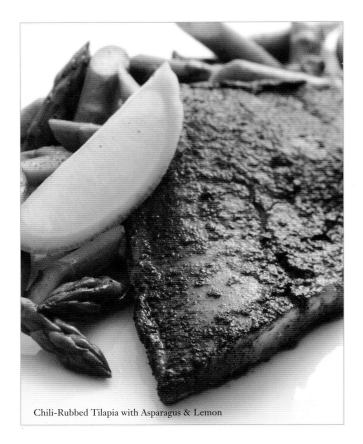

Chili-Rubbed Tilapia with Asparagus & Lemon

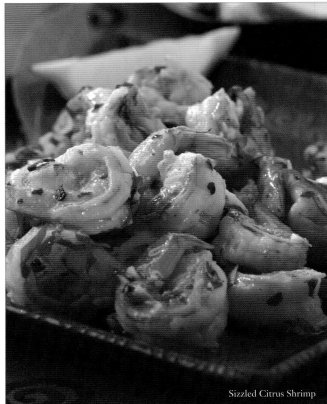

Sizzled Citrus Shrimp

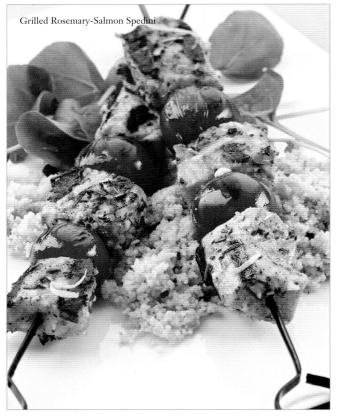

Grilled Rosemary-Salmon Spedini

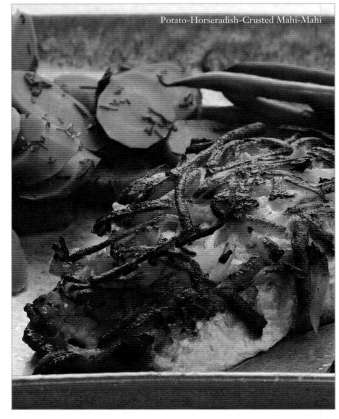

Potato-Horseradish-Crusted Mahi-Mahi

FISH & SEAFOOD

“ Ruling a large kingdom is like cooking a small fish;
handle gently and never overdo it. **”**

LAO-TZU, CHINESE PHILOSOPHER (6TH CENTURY B.C.)

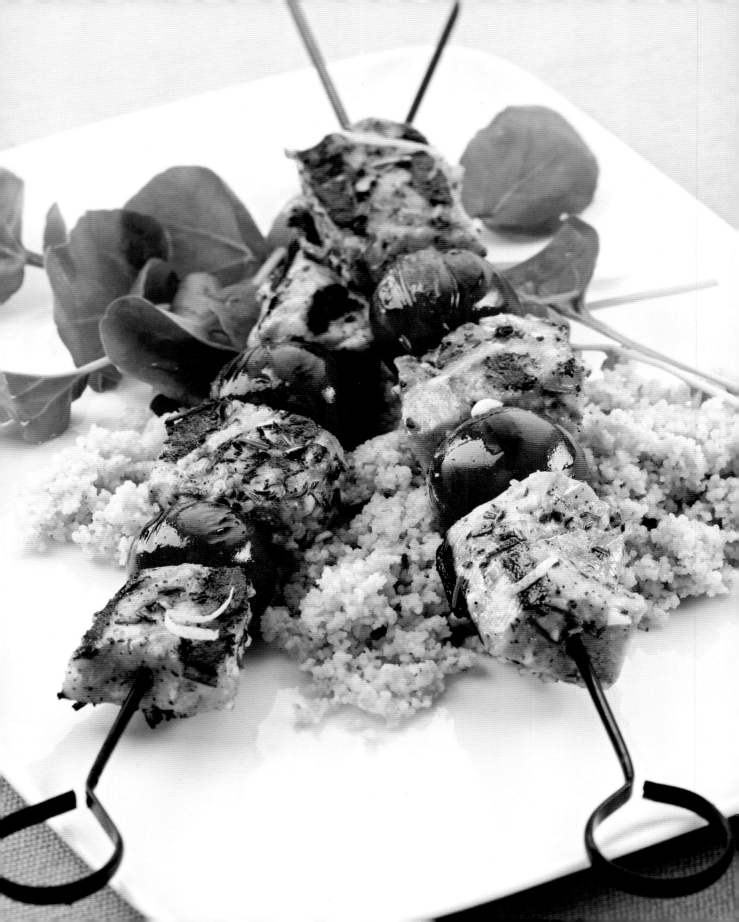

GRILLED ROSEMARY-SALMON SPEDINI

If you can find (or grow) them, use sturdy rosemary branches, stripped of leaves, as skewers for these Italian kebabs; they'll add a subtle, smoky flavor that hints of pine. Oil your grill well to prevent sticking, don't move the kebabs around unnecessarily and keep a close eye on the fire to avoid flare-ups.

- 2   teaspoons minced fresh rosemary
- 2   teaspoons extra-virgin olive oil
- 2   cloves garlic, minced
- 1   teaspoon freshly grated lemon zest
- 1   teaspoon lemon juice
- ½   teaspoon kosher salt
- ¼   teaspoon freshly ground pepper
- 1   pound center-cut salmon fillet, skinned (*see Tip, page 245*) and cut into 1-inch cubes
- 1   pint cherry tomatoes

1. Preheat grill to medium-high.
2. Combine rosemary, oil, garlic, lemon zest, lemon juice, salt and pepper in a medium bowl. Add salmon; toss to coat. Alternating the salmon and tomatoes, divide among eight 12-inch skewers.
3. Oil the grill rack (*see Tip, page 245*). Grill the spedini, carefully turning once, until the salmon is cooked through, 4 to 6 minutes total. Serve immediately.

MAKES 4 SERVINGS, 2 SKEWERS EACH.

PER SERVING:

246 CALORIES

15 g fat (3 g sat, 6 g mono)
67 mg cholesterol
4 g carbohydrate
23 g protein
1 g fiber
211 mg sodium
598 mg potassium

NUTRITION BONUS:
Selenium (60% daily value)
Vitamin C (25% dv)
Potassium (17% dv)
Vitamin A (15% dv)
Excellent source of omega-3s

Healthy ♓ Weight

Lower ⬇ Carbs

ACTIVE TIME: **30 MINUTES**

TOTAL: **30 MINUTES**

TO MAKE AHEAD: **Prepare spedini (Step 2), cover and refrigerate for up to 8 hours. Proceed with grilling (Steps 1 & 3) when ready to serve.**

EQUIPMENT: **Eight 12-inch skewers**

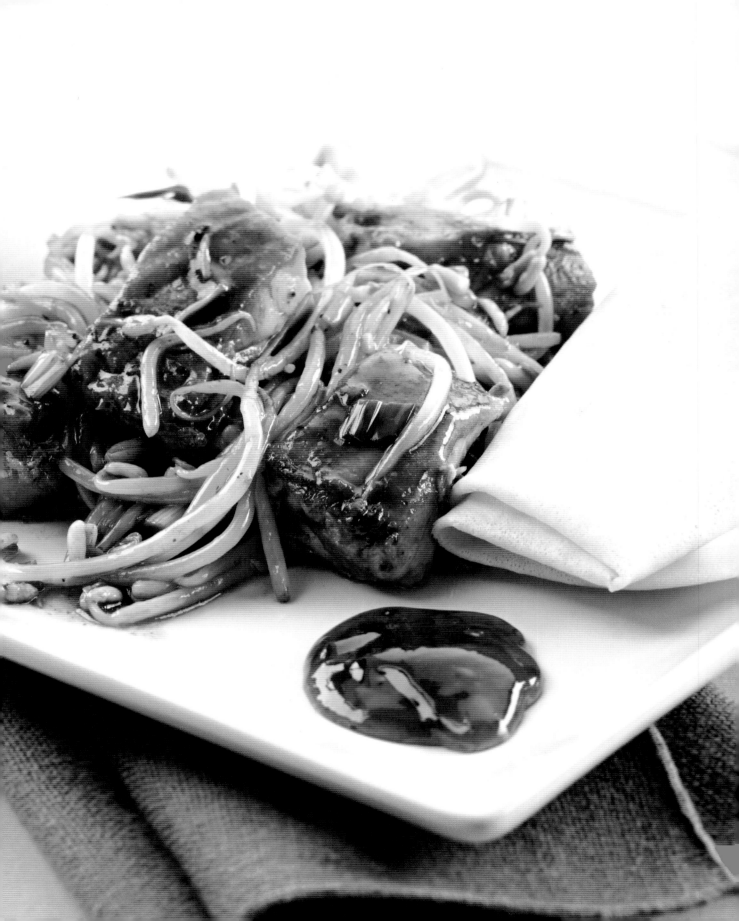

BLACK BEAN-SALMON STIR-FRY

Add bean sprouts to your list of vegetables to explore and appreciate. They're loaded with fiber and vitamin C, and the generous amount in this stir-fry gives it an appealing texture.

- ¼ cup water
- 2 tablespoons rice vinegar
- 2 tablespoons black bean-garlic sauce (*see Note*)
- 1 tablespoon Shao Hsing rice wine *or* dry sherry (*see Note, page 245*)
- 2 teaspoons cornstarch
  Pinch of crushed red pepper
- 1 tablespoon canola oil
- 1 pound salmon, skinned (*see Tip, page 245*) and cut into 1-inch cubes
- 12 ounces mung bean sprouts (6 cups)
- 1 bunch scallions, sliced

1. Whisk water, vinegar, black bean-garlic sauce, rice wine (or sherry), cornstarch and crushed red pepper in a small bowl until combined.
2. Heat oil in a large nonstick skillet over medium-high heat. Add salmon and cook, stirring gently, for 2 minutes. Add bean sprouts, scallions and the sauce mixture (the pan will be full). Cook, stirring, until the sprouts are cooked down and tender, 2 to 3 minutes.

MAKES 4 SERVINGS, ABOUT 1 ½ CUPS EACH.

PER SERVING:

302 CALORIES

17 g fat (3 g sat, 6 g mono)
67 mg cholesterol
12 g carbohydrate
26 g protein
3 g fiber
802 mg sodium
608 mg potassium

NUTRITION BONUS:
Selenium (60% daily value)
Vitamin C (33% dv)
Folate (24% dv)
Potassium (17% dv)
Excellent source of omega-3s

Healthy ⚖ Weight

Lower ⬇ Carbs

ACTIVE TIME: **20 MINUTES**

TOTAL: **20 MINUTES**

INGREDIENT NOTE:

- Black bean-garlic sauce, a savory, salty sauce used in Chinese cooking, is made from fermented black beans, garlic and rice wine. Find it in the Asian-foods section of some supermarkets or at Asian markets.

MUSTARD-CRUSTED SALMON

This updated bistro classic makes a simple yet sophisticated dinner any night of the week. You might want to consider doubling the batch and using the remaining salmon in a tossed salad for the next day's meal.

1 ¼	pounds center-cut salmon fillets, cut into 4 portions
¼	teaspoon salt, or to taste
	Freshly ground pepper to taste
¼	cup reduced-fat sour cream
2	tablespoons stone-ground mustard
2	teaspoons lemon juice
	Lemon wedges

1. Preheat broiler. Line a broiler pan or baking sheet with foil, then coat it with cooking spray.

2. Place salmon pieces, skin-side down, on the prepared pan. Season with salt and pepper. Combine sour cream, mustard and lemon juice in a small bowl. Spread evenly over the salmon.

3. Broil the salmon 5 inches from the heat source until it is opaque in the center, 10 to 12 minutes. Serve with lemon wedges.

MAKES 4 SERVINGS.

SAUTÉED SOLE WITH ORANGE-SHALLOT SAUCE

Sole (or other mild white fish like halibut) is ideal for time-strapped cooks with healthy intentions; it's mild-flavored, lean and ready in minutes. Choose Pacific varieties as Atlantic sole is becoming overfished. A large nonstick skillet is highly recommended. Otherwise, cook the fillets in two batches, using 1½ teaspoons oil per batch.

- ⅓ cup all-purpose flour
- ½ teaspoon salt, or to taste
  Freshly ground pepper to taste
- 1 pound Pacific sole *or* Pacific halibut fillets
- 1 tablespoon extra-virgin olive oil
- 1 large shallot, finely chopped (about ⅓ cup)
- ½ cup dry white wine
- 1 cup freshly squeezed orange juice
- 2 heaping teaspoons Dijon mustard
- 2 teaspoons butter
- 2 tablespoons chopped fresh parsley

1. Mix flour, salt and pepper in a shallow dish. Thoroughly dredge fish fillets in the mixture.

2. Heat oil in a large nonstick skillet over medium-high heat until shimmering but not smoking. Add the fish and cook until lightly browned and just opaque in the center, 3 to 4 minutes per side. Transfer to a plate and cover loosely with foil.

3. Add shallot to the pan and cook over medium-high heat, stirring often, until softened and beginning to brown, about 3 minutes. Add wine and bring to a simmer, scraping up any browned bits. Cook until most of the liquid has evaporated, 1 to 2 minutes. Add orange juice and mustard; bring to a boil. Reduce heat to low and simmer until the sauce thickens a bit, about 5 minutes. Add butter and parsley; stir until the butter has melted. Transfer fish to individual plates, top with sauce and serve.

MAKES 4 SERVINGS.

PER SERVING:

222 CALORIES

7 g fat (2 g sat, 3 g mono)

59 mg cholesterol

12 g carbohydrate

23 g protein

0 g fiber

237 mg sodium

612 mg potassium

NUTRITION BONUS:
Vitamin C (60% daily value)
Potassium (31% dv)
Folate (20% dv)

Healthy ⚥ Weight

Lower ⬇ Carbs

ACTIVE TIME: **30 MINUTES**

TOTAL: **30 MINUTES**

AT THE FISH COUNTER

- When buying fish, trust your instincts. Look for red gills, bright reflective skin, firm flesh, an undamaged layer of scales and no browning anywhere. The smell should be sweet, like a morning on the beach. The best whole fish look alive, as if they just came out of the water.

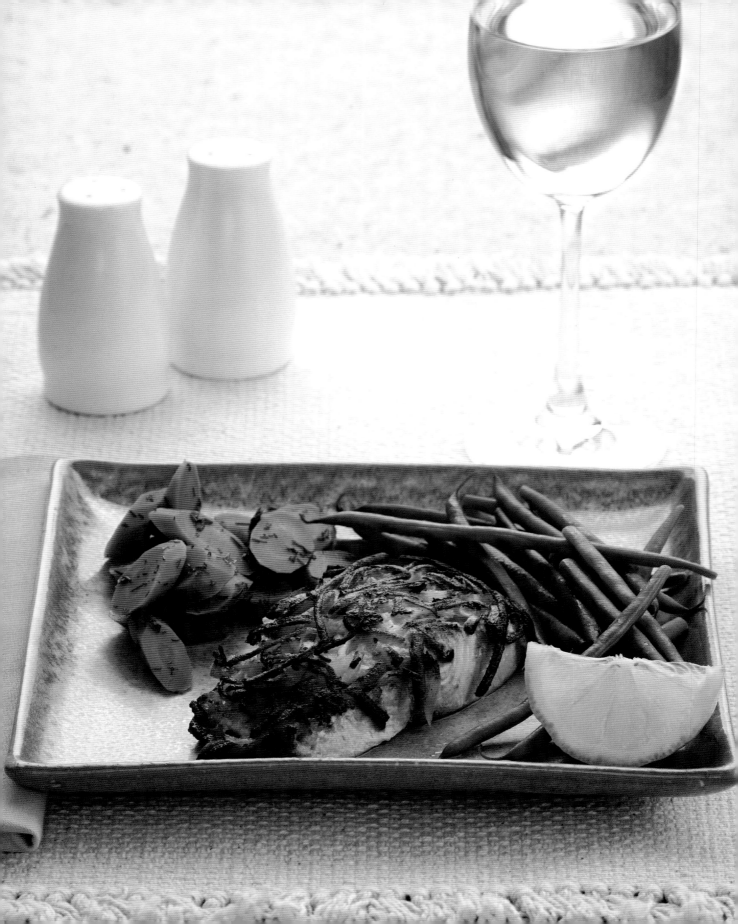

POTATO-HORSERADISH-CRUSTED MAHI-MAHI

With precooked shredded potatoes, this chef-worthy dish takes only minutes to assemble. Try it with steamed carrots and green beans tossed with a little olive oil and snipped fresh dill.

1	cup precooked shredded potatoes (*see Note*)
1	shallot, finely chopped
1	tablespoon prepared horseradish
1	teaspoon Dijon mustard
1/2	teaspoon garlic salt
1/4	teaspoon freshly ground pepper
1 1/4	pounds mahi-mahi, skin removed, cut into 4 portions
4	teaspoons reduced-fat mayonnaise
1	tablespoon canola oil
1	lemon, quartered

1. Combine potatoes, shallot, horseradish, mustard, garlic salt and pepper in a medium bowl. Spread each portion of fish with 1 teaspoon mayonnaise, then top with one-fourth of the potato mixture, pressing the mixture onto the fish.

2. Heat oil in a large nonstick skillet over medium-high heat. Carefully place the fish in the pan potato-side down and cook until crispy and browned, 4 to 5 minutes. Gently turn the fish over, reduce the heat to medium and continue cooking until the fish flakes easily with a fork, 4 to 5 minutes more. Serve with lemon wedges.

MAKES 4 SERVINGS.

PER SERVING:

205 CALORIES

6 g fat (1 g sat, 3 g mono)

105 mg cholesterol

9 g carbohydrate

27 g protein

1 g fiber

311 mg sodium

623 mg potassium

NUTRITION BONUS:
Selenium (74% daily value)
Potassium (18% dv)

Healthy)(Weight

Lower ⬇ Carbs

ACTIVE TIME: **25 MINUTES**

TOTAL: **25 MINUTES**

INGREDIENT NOTE:

- Look for precooked shredded potatoes in the refrigerated section of the produce department—near other fresh prepared vegetables.

210 CALORIES

10 g fat (1 g sat, 6 g mono)

48 mg cholesterol

8 g carbohydrate

24 g protein

4 g fiber

418 mg sodium

645 mg potassium

NUTRITION BONUS:
Vitamin C (37% daily value)
Folate (33% dv)
Iron (33% dv)
Fiber (24% dv)

Healthy)(Weight

Lower ⬇ Carbs

ACTIVE TIME: **20 MINUTES**

TOTAL: **20 MINUTES**

CHILI-RUBBED TILAPIA WITH ASPARAGUS & LEMON

Tilapia, an ocean-friendly fish, has a pleasant, mild flavor. It's great with a spice rub, a familiar flavoring technique that works equally as well on the grill or in a pan. You could also use this rub on chicken breasts or toss it with lightly oiled shrimp before cooking.

> 2 pounds asparagus, tough ends trimmed, cut into 1-inch pieces
> 2 tablespoons chili powder
> ½ teaspoon garlic powder
> ½ teaspoon salt, divided
> 1 pound tilapia, Pacific sole *or* other firm white fish fillets
> 2 tablespoons extra-virgin olive oil
> 3 tablespoons lemon juice

1. Bring 1 inch of water to a boil in a large saucepan. Put asparagus in a steamer basket, place in the pan, cover and steam until tender-crisp, about 4 minutes. Transfer to a large plate, spreading out to cool.

2. Combine chili powder, garlic powder and ¼ teaspoon salt on a plate. Dredge fillets in the spice mixture to coat. Heat oil in a large nonstick skillet over medium-high heat. Add the fish and cook until just opaque in the center, gently turning halfway, 5 to 7 minutes total. Divide among 4 plates. Immediately add lemon juice, the remaining ¼ teaspoon salt and asparagus to the pan and cook, stirring constantly, until the asparagus is coated and heated through, about 2 minutes. Serve the asparagus with the fish.

MAKES **4** SERVINGS.

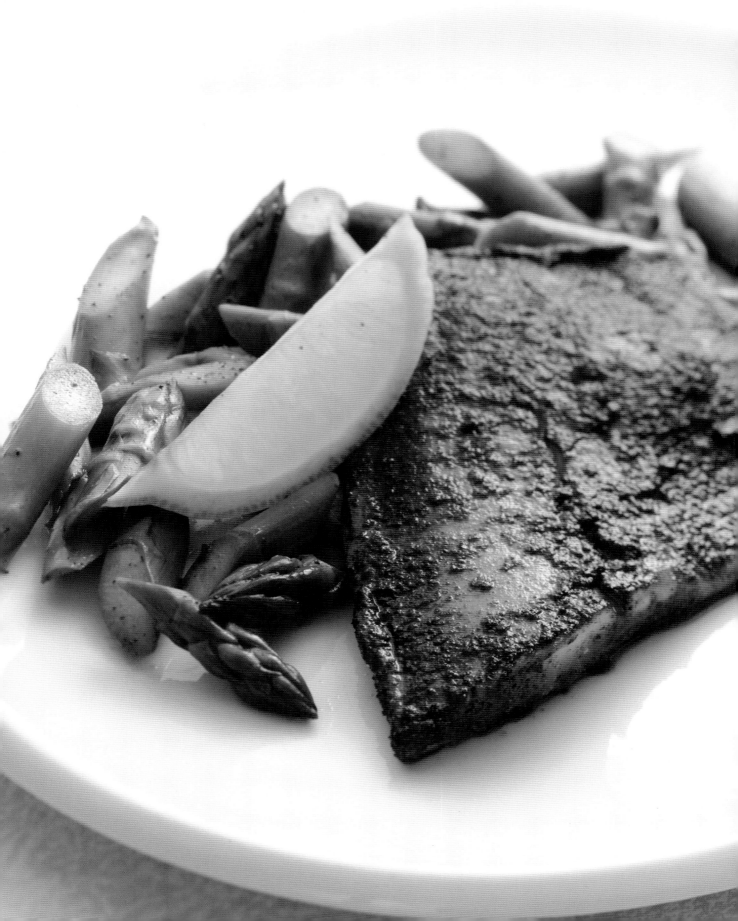

245 CALORIES

8 g fat (1 g sat, 6 g mono)

115 mg cholesterol

26 g carbohydrate

23 g protein

8 g fiber

596 mg sodium

855 mg potassium

NUTRITION BONUS:
Selenium (43% daily value)
Fiber (33% dv)
Vitamin C (30% dv)
Iron (25% dv)
Potassium (24% dv)
Vitamin A (20% dv)

Healthy)(Weight

High ⬆ Fiber

ACTIVE TIME: **30 MINUTES**

TOTAL: **30 MINUTES**

INGREDIENT NOTE:

■ When you use canned beans in a recipe, be sure to rinse them first in a colander under cold running water, as their canning liquid often contains a fair amount of sodium.

PAPRIKA SHRIMP & GREEN BEAN SAUTÉ

Crisp-tender beans add snap and color to the garlicky melange of shrimp and creamy butter beans in this Spanish-inspired sauté. Prepeeled shrimp can be worth the extra cost for the amount of time they'll save on a harried weeknight. (Photograph: front cover.)

4	cups green beans, trimmed (about 12 ounces)
3	tablespoons extra-virgin olive oil
¼	cup minced garlic
2	teaspoons paprika
1	pound raw shrimp (21-25 per pound), peeled and deveined
2	16-ounce cans large butter beans *or* cannellini beans, rinsed (*see Note*)
¼	cup sherry vinegar *or* red-wine vinegar
½	cup chopped fresh parsley, divided
	Freshly ground pepper to taste

1. Bring 1 inch of water to a boil in a large saucepan. Put green beans in a steamer basket, place in the pan, cover and steam until tender-crisp, 4 to 6 minutes.

2. Meanwhile, heat oil in a large skillet over medium-high heat. Add garlic and paprika and cook, stirring constantly, until just fragrant but not browned, about 20 seconds. Add shrimp and cook until pink and opaque, about 2 minutes per side. Stir in butter beans (or cannellini) and vinegar; cook, stirring occasionally, until heated through, about 2 minutes. Stir in ¼ cup parsley.

3. Divide the green beans among 4 plates. Top with the shrimp mixture. Sprinkle with pepper and the remaining ¼ cup parsley.

MAKES **6** SERVINGS.

SHRIMP WITH BROCCOLI

Here's an example of international cooking at its fastest and best: a speedy Asian favorite, that can be prepared in less time than it takes to get takeout.

- ⅔ cup bottled clam juice *or* reduced-sodium chicken broth
- 1 teaspoon cornstarch
- 1 tablespoon minced garlic, divided
- 3 teaspoons extra-virgin olive oil, divided
- ¼-½ teaspoon crushed red pepper
- 1 pound raw shrimp (21-25 per pound), peeled and deveined
- ¼ teaspoon salt, divided
- 4 cups broccoli florets
- ⅔ cup water
- 2 tablespoons chopped fresh basil
- 1 teaspoon lemon juice
  Freshly ground pepper to taste
  Lemon wedges

1. Combine clam juice (or broth), cornstarch and half the garlic in a small bowl; whisk until smooth. Set aside.

2. Heat 1½ teaspoons oil in a large nonstick skillet over medium-high heat. Add the remaining garlic and crushed red pepper to taste; cook, stirring, until fragrant but not browned, about 30 seconds. Add shrimp and ⅛ teaspoon salt. Sauté until the shrimp are pink, about 3 minutes. Transfer to a bowl.

3. Add the remaining 1½ teaspoons oil to the pan. Add broccoli and the remaining ⅛ teaspoon salt; cook, stirring, for 1 minute. Add water, cover and cook until the broccoli is crisp-tender, about 3 minutes. Transfer to the bowl with the shrimp.

4. Add the reserved clam juice mixture to the pan and cook, stirring, over medium-high heat, until thickened, 3 to 4 minutes. Stir in basil and season with lemon juice and pepper. Add the shrimp and broccoli; heat through. Serve immediately, with lemon wedges.

MAKES 4 SERVINGS, 1½ CUPS EACH.

PER SERVING:

178 CALORIES

6 g fat (1 g sat, 3 g mono)
172 mg cholesterol
6 g carbohydrate
25 g protein
2 g fiber
520 mg sodium
459 mg potassium

NUTRITION BONUS:
Vitamin C (120% daily value)
Selenium (65% dv)
Vitamin A (50% dv)
Iron (20% dv)

Healthy ⚖ Weight

Lower ⬇ Carbs

ACTIVE TIME: **25 MINUTES**

TOTAL: **25 MINUTES**

SHOPPING TIP:

- Shrimp are sold by the number needed to make one pound—for example, "21-25 count" or "31-40 count"—and by more generic size names, such as "large" or "extra large." Size names don't always correspond to the actual "count size." To be sure you're getting the size you want, order by the count (or number) per pound.

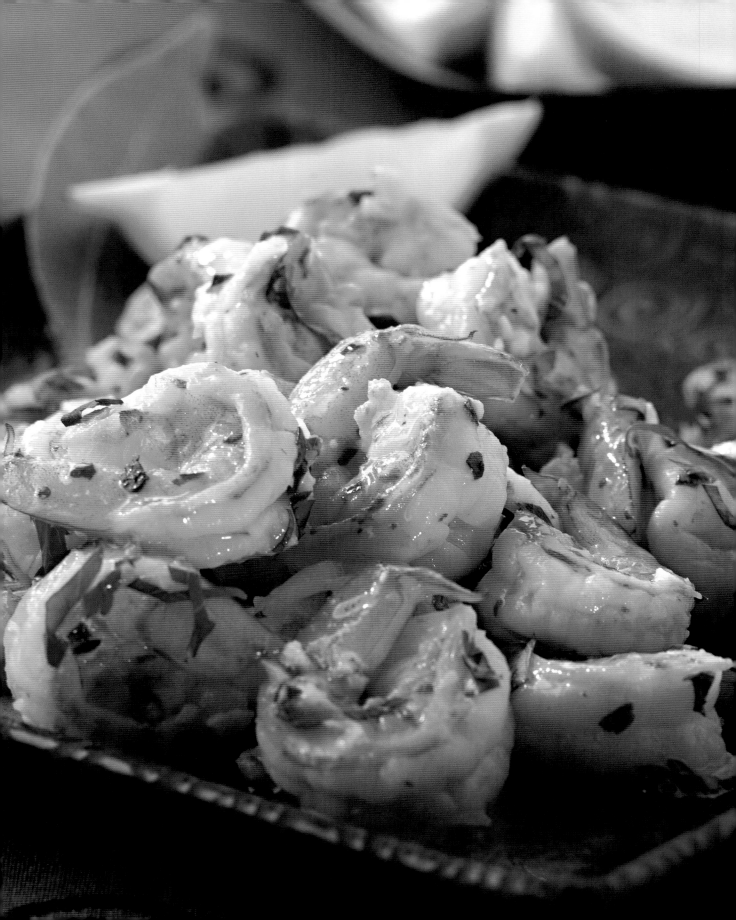

SIZZLED CITRUS SHRIMP

This super-fast sauté is a lesson in simplicity: all shrimp really needs to dazzle is lots of garlic and a splash of lemon. Serve it with whole-wheat couscous and sugar snap peas, steamed tender-crisp.

MARINADE & SHRIMP

- 3   tablespoons lemon juice
- 3   tablespoons dry white wine
- 2   teaspoons extra-virgin olive oil
- 3   cloves garlic, minced
- 1   pound medium shrimp (30-40 per pound), peeled and deveined

SAUCE

- 1   teaspoon extra-virgin olive oil
- 1   bay leaf
- 1/4   teaspoon crushed red pepper
- 1/4   teaspoon salt, or to taste
- 2   tablespoons chopped fresh parsley

1. Combine lemon juice, wine, 2 teaspoons oil and garlic in a medium bowl. Add shrimp and toss to coat. Cover and marinate in the refrigerator for 15 minutes, tossing occasionally. Drain well, reserving marinade.

2. Heat 1 teaspoon oil in a 12-inch nonstick skillet over medium-high heat. Add shrimp and cook, turning once, until barely pink, about 30 seconds per side; transfer to a plate. Add bay leaf, crushed red pepper and the reserved marinade to the pan; simmer for 4 minutes. Return the shrimp and any accumulated juices to the pan; heat through. Season with salt, sprinkle with parsley and serve immediately.

MAKES 4 SERVINGS, ABOUT 3/4 CUP EACH.

PER SERVING:

171 CALORIES

6 g fat (1 g sat, 3 g mono)

172 mg cholesterol

4 g carbohydrate

23 g protein

1 g fiber

315 mg sodium

270 mg potassium

NUTRITION BONUS:
Vitamin A (15% daily value)
Vitamin C (15% dv)

Healthy)(Weight

Lower ⬇ Carbs

ACTIVE TIME: **15 MINUTES**
(including peeling shrimp)

TOTAL: **40 MINUTES**

PER SERVING:

210 CALORIES

4 g fat (0 g sat, 0 g mono)

182 mg cholesterol

33 g carbohydrate

17 g protein

11 g fiber

928 mg sodium

103 mg potassium

NUTRITION BONUS:
Vitamin A (35% daily value)
Zinc (30% dv)
Magnesium (22% dv)
Calcium (20% dv)
Vitamin C (15% dv)

Healthy)((Weight

High ⬆ Fiber

ACTIVE TIME: **10 MINUTES**

TOTAL: **10 MINUTES**

SHRIMP LOUIS SALAD SANDWICH

This sandwich is a spin on the West Coast classic Louis salad—normally a big helping of fresh crab or shrimp served atop a cool pile of iceberg lettuce and doused with a heavy Russian-like dressing, known as Louis sauce. We've turned it into a healthy sandwich with lean seafood and a tangy, lighter Louis dressing. Crab would also be excellent on this sandwich—for convenience you can buy it in a 3¹/2-ounce pouch near the canned fish at the supermarket.

2   3-ounce pouches gulf shrimp, drained
1   tablespoon ketchup
1   tablespoon reduced-fat mayonnaise
1   tablespoon dill relish *or* minced dill pickle
4   slices toasted whole-grain bread
1   cup shredded romaine lettuce *or* spinach

Mix shrimp with ketchup, mayonnaise and relish (or pickle) in a small bowl. Divide between 2 slices of bread, top with lettuce (or spinach) and the remaining bread.

MAKES **2** SERVINGS.

CRAB CAKE BURGERS

These easy burgers have a true crab flavor that isn't masked by fillers or strong seasoning. The recipe works best with convenient pasteurized crabmeat, usually found in the refrigerated case near the fish counter. We like to use the more economical claw meat, but if you prefer lump crabmeat, cut it into small, uniform pieces.

1	pound crabmeat
1	egg, lightly beaten
½	cup panko breadcrumbs (*see Note*)
¼	cup reduced-fat mayonnaise
2	tablespoons minced chives
1	tablespoon Dijon mustard
1	tablespoon lemon juice
1	teaspoon celery seed
1	teaspoon onion powder
¼	teaspoon freshly ground pepper
4	dashes hot sauce, such as Tabasco, or to taste
1	tablespoon extra-virgin olive oil
2	teaspoons unsalted butter

1. Mix crab, egg, breadcrumbs, mayonnaise, chives, mustard, lemon juice, celery seed, onion powder, pepper and hot sauce in a large bowl. Form into 6 patties.

2. Heat oil and butter in a large nonstick skillet over medium heat until the butter stops foaming. Cook the patties until golden brown, about 4 minutes per side.

MAKES **6** SERVINGS.

PER SERVING:

161 CALORIES

8 g fat (2 g sat, 3 g mono)
86 mg cholesterol
6 g carbohydrate
16 g protein
0 g fiber
350 mg sodium
293 mg potassium

NUTRITION BONUS:
Selenium (44% daily value)
Zinc (20% dv)
Vitamin C (15% dv)

Healthy ⋊⋉ Weight

Lower ⬇ Carbs

ACTIVE TIME: **20 MINUTES**

TOTAL: **20 MINUTES**

INGREDIENT NOTE:

- Panko breadcrumbs, also known as Japanese breadcrumbs or bread flakes, are coarser in texture than other dried breadcrumbs. They produce a crispy crust and are less likely to become soggy than finely ground breadcrumbs. Look for panko in the Asian food section of large supermarkets and in specialty Asian markets.

264 CALORIES

7 g fat (3 g sat, 1 g mono)

68 mg cholesterol

19 g carbohydrate

31 g protein

3 g fiber

403 mg sodium

274 mg potassium

NUTRITION BONUS:
Vitamin A (20% daily value)
Vitamin C (20% dv)

Healthy ⅜ Weight

Lower ↓ Carbs

ACTIVE TIME: **10 MINUTES**

TOTAL: **15 MINUTES**

INGREDIENT NOTE:

- Canned white tuna comes from the large albacore and can be high in mercury content. Chunk light, on the other hand, which comes from smaller fish, skipjack or yellowfin, is best for health-conscious eaters.

THE EATINGWELL TUNA MELT

The secret to a healthier tuna melt? Just add plenty of vegetables, use a light hand with the mayonnaise—and shred the sharp, flavorful cheese so a little goes a long way. You'll still get a powerful cheese "hit" in every gooey, satisfying bite.

4	slices whole-wheat bread
2	6-ounce cans chunk light tuna (*see Note*), drained
1	medium shallot, minced (2 tablespoons)
2	tablespoons reduced-fat mayonnaise
1	tablespoon lemon juice
1	tablespoon minced flat-leaf parsley
⅛	teaspoon salt
	Dash of hot sauce, such as Tabasco
	Freshly ground pepper to taste
2	tomatoes, sliced
½	cup shredded sharp Cheddar cheese

1. Preheat the broiler.
2. Toast bread in a toaster.
3. Combine tuna, shallot, mayonnaise, lemon juice, parsley, salt, hot sauce and pepper in a medium bowl. Spread ¼ cup of the tuna mixture on each slice of toast; top with tomato slices and 2 tablespoons cheese. Place sandwiches on a baking sheet and broil until the cheese is bubbling and golden brown, 3 to 5 minutes. Serve immediately.

MAKES **4** SERVINGS.

TUSCAN-STYLE TUNA SALAD

This streamlined version of a northern Italian idea is perfect for a summer evening: no-fuss, no-cook and big taste. You can even make it ahead and store it, covered, in the refrigerator for several days. If you do, use it as a wrap filling for the next day's lunch.

2	6-ounce cans chunk light tuna, drained
1	15-ounce can small white beans, such as cannellini *or* great northern, rinsed
10	cherry tomatoes, quartered
4	scallions, trimmed and sliced
2	tablespoons extra-virgin olive oil
2	tablespoons lemon juice
1/4	teaspoon salt
	Freshly ground pepper to taste

Combine tuna, beans, tomatoes, scallions, oil, lemon juice, salt and pepper in a medium bowl. Stir gently. Refrigerate until ready to serve.

MAKES 4 SERVINGS, 1 CUP EACH.

PER SERVING:

253 CALORIES

8 g fat (1 g sat, 5 g mono)
53 mg cholesterol
20 g carbohydrate
31 g protein
6 g fiber
453 mg sodium
451 mg potassium

NUTRITION BONUS:
Fiber (25% daily value)
Vitamin C (20% dv)

Healthy)(Weight

Lower ⬇ Carbs

High ⬆ Fiber

ACTIVE TIME: **10 MINUTES**

TOTAL: **10 MINUTES**

TO MAKE AHEAD: **Cover and refrigerate for up to 2 days.**

EASY LUNCH IDEA

CRACKERS & TUNA

Healthy)(Weight   Lower ⬇ Carbs

Top 2 multigrain crispbread crackers, such as Wasa, with 2 tablespoons reduced-fat cream cheese, one 3-ounce can water-packed chunk light tuna and 1 sliced scallion. Squeeze a wedge of lemon on top and season with freshly ground pepper to taste.

MAKES 1 SERVING.

PER SERVING: 229 CALORIES; 6 g fat (4 g sat, 2 g mono); 42 mg cholesterol; 15 g carbohydrate; 27 g protein; 1 g fiber; 382 mg sodium; 356 mg potassium.
NUTRITION BONUS: Selenium (100% daily value), Iron & Vitamin C (15% dv).

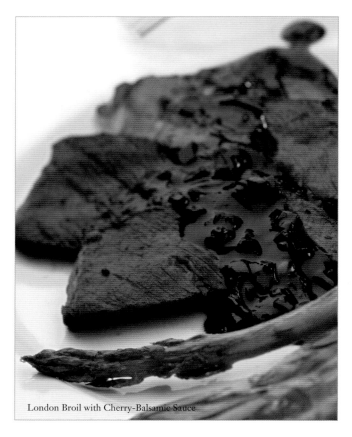

London Broil with Cherry-Balsamic Sauce

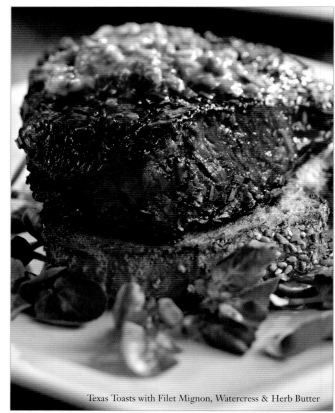

Texas Toasts with Filet Mignon, Watercress & Herb Butter

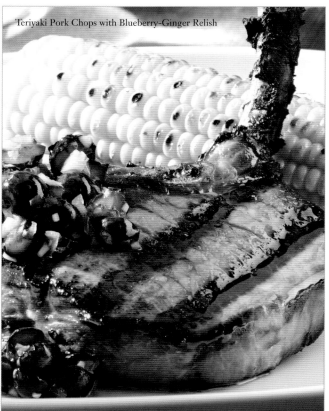

Teriyaki Pork Chops with Blueberry-Ginger Relish

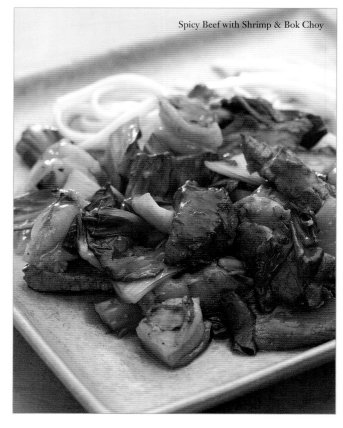

Spicy Beef with Shrimp & Bok Choy

BEEF & PORK

❝Vegetables are interesting but lack a sense of purpose
when unaccompanied by a good cut of meat.❞

FRAN LEBOWITZ, HUMORIST

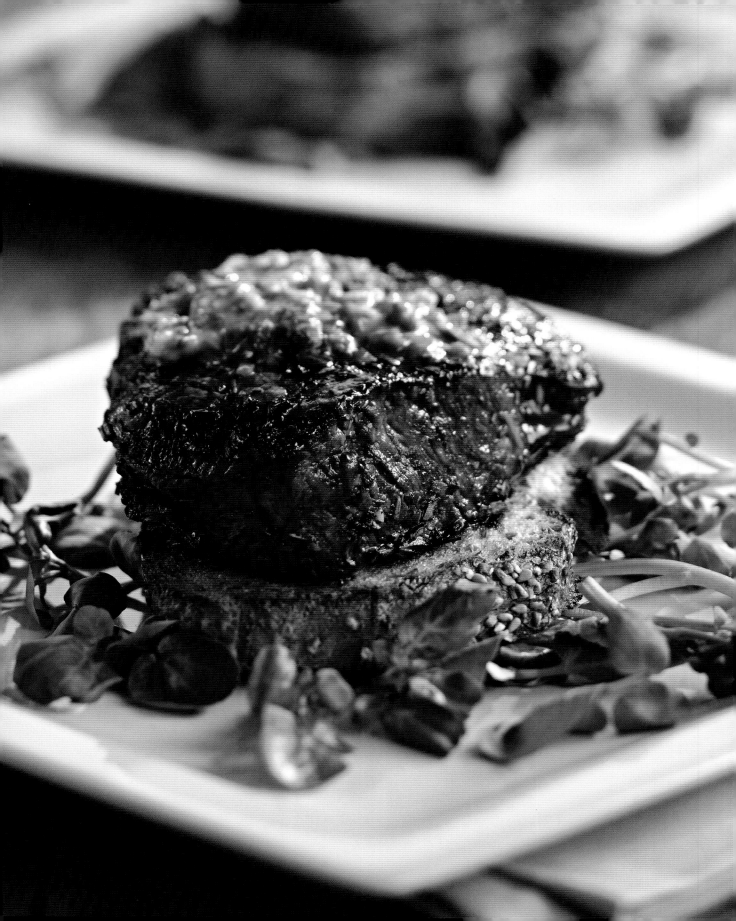

TEXAS TOASTS WITH FILET MIGNON, WATERCRESS & HERB BUTTER

Yes, a juicy grilled steak and even a bit of wonderful, herb-flecked butter can fit into your healthy eating plans; this soul-satisfying meal is a case in point. Make a double batch of the butter to keep in the freezer for jazzing up future grilled entrees like pork chops, chicken breasts or fish (a little goes a long way).

1	tablespoon whipped *or* regular butter, slightly softened
3	teaspoons extra-virgin olive oil, divided
1	tablespoon minced chives *or* shallot
1	tablespoon capers, rinsed and chopped
3	teaspoons minced fresh marjoram *or* oregano, divided
1	teaspoon freshly grated lemon zest, divided
1	teaspoon lemon juice
¾	teaspoon kosher salt, divided
½	teaspoon freshly ground pepper, divided
1	tablespoon minced fresh rosemary
1	clove garlic, minced, plus 1 clove garlic, peeled and halved
1	pound filet mignon, about 1 ½ inches thick, trimmed of fat and cut into 4 portions
4	slices whole-grain bread
4	cups watercress, trimmed and chopped

1. Preheat grill to high.

2. Mash butter in a small bowl with the back of a spoon until it's soft and creamy. Stir in 2 teaspoons oil until combined. Add chives (or shallot), capers, 1 teaspoon marjoram (or oregano), ½ teaspoon lemon zest, lemon juice, ½ teaspoon salt and ¼ teaspoon pepper. Cover and place in the freezer to chill.

3. Combine the remaining 1 teaspoon oil, remaining 2 teaspoons marjoram (or oregano), remaining ½ teaspoon lemon zest, remaining ¼ teaspoon salt and pepper, rosemary and minced garlic in a small bowl. Rub on both sides of steak. Rub both sides of bread with the halved garlic clove; discard the garlic.

4. Grill the steak 3 to 5 minutes per side for medium-rare. Grill the bread until toasted, 30 seconds to 1 minute per side. Transfer the toasts to a large plate, place the steaks on top of the toasts and spread the herb butter on top of the steaks; let rest for 5 minutes. Divide watercress among 4 plates and top with the steak-topped toasts.

MAKES 4 SERVINGS.

PER SERVING:

303 CALORIES

14 g fat (5 g sat, 6 g mono)

80 mg cholesterol

15 g carbohydrate

29 g protein

5 g fiber

438 mg sodium

462 mg potassium

NUTRITION BONUS:
Zinc (46% daily value)
Selenium (44% dv)
Vitamin C (28% dv)
Iron (17% dv)

Healthy)(Weight

Lower ⬇ Carbs

High ⬆ Fiber

ACTIVE TIME: **45 MINUTES**

TOTAL: **45 MINUTES**

TO MAKE AHEAD: **Prepare herb butter (Step 2), wrap in plastic wrap and freeze for up to 1 month.**

252 CALORIES

12 g fat (4 g sat, 6 g mono)

97 mg cholesterol

5 g carbohydrate

29 g protein

0 g fiber

172 mg sodium

286 mg potassium

NUTRITION BONUS:
Zinc (27% daily value)
Iron (15% dv)

Healthy ⅓⅔ Weight

Lower ⬇ Carbs

ACTIVE TIME: **45 MINUTES**

TOTAL: **3¼ HOURS**

SHOPPING TIP:

■ Although it is not the leanest cut of beef, chuck is still our choice for pot roast because it doesn't dry out during braising. You will find pockets of fat as you carve it, but they are easy to remove.

COFFEE-BRAISED POT ROAST WITH CARAMELIZED ONIONS

We've always had a soft spot for pot roast made with onion-soup mix, but dread its excessive sodium content. This recipe starts with caramelized onions instead, and deepens the flavors with rich-tasting (but calorie-free) coffee and balsamic vinegar.

1	4-pound beef chuck roast (*see Tip*), trimmed of fat
½	teaspoon salt, or to taste
	Freshly ground pepper to taste
4	teaspoons extra-virgin olive oil, divided
2	large onions, halved and thinly sliced (4 cups)
4	cloves garlic, minced
1	teaspoon dried thyme
¾	cup strong brewed coffee
2	tablespoons balsamic vinegar
2	tablespoons cornstarch mixed with 2 tablespoons water

1. Preheat oven to 300°F.

2. Season beef with salt and pepper. Heat 2 teaspoons oil in a Dutch oven or soup pot over medium-high heat. Add beef and cook, turning from time to time, until well browned on all sides, 5 to 7 minutes. Transfer to a plate.

3. Add the remaining 2 teaspoons oil to the pot. Add onions, reduce heat to medium and cook, stirring often, until softened and golden, 5 to 7 minutes. Add garlic and thyme; cook, stirring, for 1 minute. Stir in coffee and vinegar; bring to a simmer. Return the beef to the pot and spoon some onions over it. Cover and transfer to the oven.

4. Braise the beef in the oven until fork-tender but not falling apart, 2½ to 3 hours. Transfer beef to a cutting board, tent with foil and let rest for about 10 minutes.

5. Meanwhile, skim fat from the braising liquid; bring to a boil over medium-high heat. Add the cornstarch mixture and cook, whisking, until the gravy thickens slightly, about 1 minute. Season with pepper. Carve the beef and serve with gravy.

MAKES **10** SERVINGS, ABOUT **3** OUNCES MEAT & ⅓ CUP GRAVY EACH.

SOUTHWESTERN STEAK & PEPPERS

This juicy spice-crusted steak is all about big, deep flavors, thanks to a few surprise ingredients in the sauce. Slice the steak very thinly across the grain to ensure the most tender results.

- ½ teaspoon ground cumin
- ½ teaspoon ground coriander
- ½ teaspoon chili powder
- ¼ teaspoon salt, or to taste
- ¾ teaspoon coarsely ground pepper, plus more to taste
- 1 pound boneless top sirloin steak, trimmed of fat
- 3 cloves garlic, peeled, 1 halved and 2 minced
- 3 teaspoons canola oil *or* extra-virgin olive oil, divided
- 2 red bell peppers, thinly sliced
- 1 medium white onion, halved lengthwise and thinly sliced
- 1 teaspoon brown sugar
- ½ cup brewed coffee *or* prepared instant coffee
- ¼ cup balsamic vinegar
- 4 cups watercress sprigs

1. Mix cumin, coriander, chili powder, salt and ¾ teaspoon pepper in a small bowl. Rub steak with the cut garlic. Rub the spice mix all over the steak.

2. Heat 2 teaspoons oil in a large heavy skillet, preferably cast iron, over medium-high heat. Add the steak and cook to desired doneness, 4 to 6 minutes per side for medium-rare. Transfer to a cutting board and let rest.

3. Add remaining 1 teaspoon oil to the skillet. Add bell peppers and onion; cook, stirring often, until softened, about 4 minutes. Add minced garlic and brown sugar; cook, stirring often, for 1 minute. Add coffee, vinegar and any accumulated meat juices; cook for 3 minutes to intensify flavor. Season with pepper.

4. To serve, mound 1 cup watercress on each plate. Top with the sautéed peppers and onion. Slice the steak thinly across the grain and arrange on the vegetables. Pour the sauce from the pan over the steak. Serve immediately.

MAKES 4 SERVINGS.

PER SERVING:

231 CALORIES

9 g fat (2 g sat, 4 g mono)

46 mg cholesterol

12 g carbohydrate

26 g protein

3 g fiber

216 mg sodium

613 mg potassium

NUTRITION BONUS:
Vitamin C (210% daily value)
Vitamin A (60% dv)
Iron (25% dv)

Healthy)(Weight

Lower ⬇ Carbs

ACTIVE TIME: **25 MINUTES**

TOTAL: **35 MINUTES**

216 CALORIES

8 g fat (3 g sat, 3 g mono)

41 mg cholesterol

7 g carbohydrate

25 g protein

0 g fiber

260 mg sodium

429 mg potassium

NUTRITION BONUS:
Zinc (33% daily value)
Potassium (21% dv)

Healthy)(Weight

Lower ⬇ Carbs

ACTIVE TIME: **10 MINUTES**

TOTAL: **50 MINUTES**
(including marinating time)

TO MAKE AHEAD: **The meat can marinate, covered, in the refrigerator, for up to 8 hours.**

EQUIPMENT NOTE: **A ridged grill pan is great for indoor grilling, but you can also use the broiler or, if weather permits, cook the steak on an outdoor grill.**

LONDON BROIL WITH CHERRY-BALSAMIC SAUCE

"London broil" is an especially lean cut, so it benefits from the tenderizing effects of a marinade. Ours also doubles as a sauce when simmered with some shallots. Use any steak leftovers on top of a salad or in a sandwich with fresh spinach.

1/3	cup dry red wine
1/4	cup balsamic vinegar
2	tablespoons cherry preserves
2	cloves garlic, minced
1/2	teaspoon salt
	Freshly ground pepper to taste
1 1/2	pounds London broil, trimmed
3	tablespoons finely chopped shallot
1	teaspoon extra-virgin olive oil
2	teaspoons butter

1. Whisk wine, vinegar, cherry preserves, garlic, salt and pepper in a small bowl. Place meat in a shallow glass dish. Pour the marinade over the meat and turn to coat. Cover and marinate in the refrigerator, turning several times, for at least 20 minutes or up to 8 hours.

2. Remove the meat from the marinade. Pour the marinade into a small saucepan; add shallot and set aside. Brush a ridged grill pan (*see Note*) or heavy skillet with oil; heat over medium-high heat. Add the meat and cook for 10 to 12 minutes per side for medium-rare, depending on thickness, or until it reaches desired doneness. (It may appear that the meat is burning but don't worry, it will form a pleasant crust.) Transfer the meat to a cutting board; let rest for 5 minutes.

3. While the meat is cooking, bring the marinade to a boil; cook over medium-high heat for 5 to 7 minutes, or until it is reduced to about 1/2 cup. Remove from the heat; add butter and whisk until melted.

4. Slice the meat thinly against the grain. Add any juices on the cutting board to the sauce. Serve the meat with the sauce.

MAKES **6** SERVINGS.

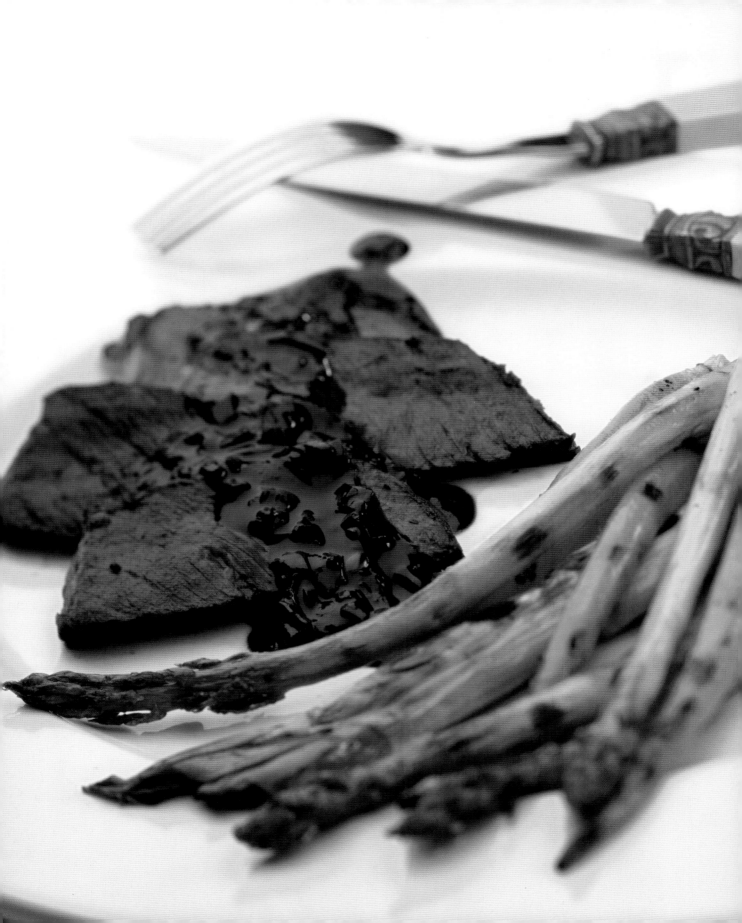

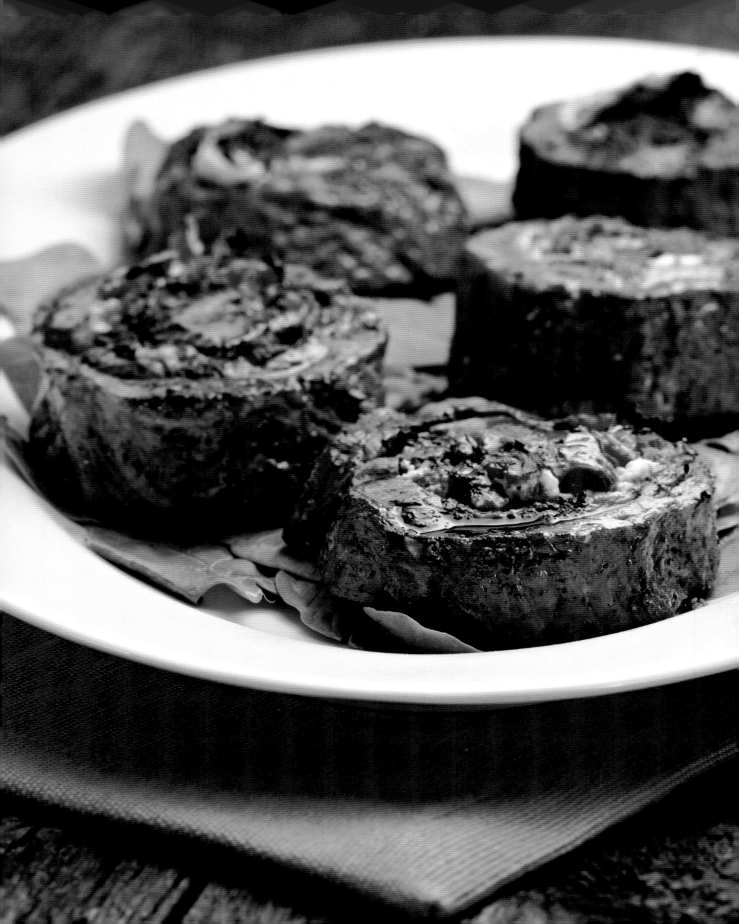

FLANK STEAK PINWHEELS

These festive wheels of steak, Boursin cheese, spinach and sun-dried tomatoes look fancy, but they're quite easy to make. For a party, arrange them on a platter atop a bed of spinach.

- ⅔ cup sun-dried tomatoes (*not* packed in oil)
- 2 cups boiling water
- 1 pound flank steak, trimmed of fat
- 1 clove garlic, minced
- 3 tablespoons light herbed cheese spread, such as Boursin (*see Variation*)
- 1 cup baby spinach
- ¾ teaspoon kosher salt
- ½ teaspoon freshly ground pepper

1. Preheat grill to high.

2. Place sun-dried tomatoes in a bowl; pour boiling water over them and let steep until softened, about 10 minutes. Drain and chop.

3. Meanwhile, place steak between 2 large pieces of plastic wrap. Pound each side of the steak thoroughly with the pointed side of a meat mallet until the steak is an even ¼-inch thickness.

4. Rub garlic all over one side of the steak. Spread cheese lengthwise in a 3-inch-wide strip down the middle of the steak. Top with the sun-dried tomatoes and spinach. Starting at one edge of a long side, roll the steak up tightly, tucking in the filling as you go.

5. Carefully rub salt and pepper all over the outside of the steak roll. Turn the roll so the overlapping edge is on top. Push 8 skewers, evenly spaced, through the roll, close to the overlapping edge to hold the roll together. Slice the roll into 8 equal portions, roughly 1 to 1½ inches thick, with a skewer in each. Lay the slices on their sides and push the skewer through so it sticks out about 1 inch.

6. Oil the grill rack (*see Tip, page 245*). Grill the pinwheels 3 to 4 minutes per side for medium-rare. Use a spatula when turning them to prevent too much filling from falling out. (Don't worry if the ends of the skewers burn. They will still hold the pinwheels together.) Remove the skewers; let the pinwheels rest for 5 minutes before serving.

MAKES 4 SERVINGS.

PER SERVING:

226 CALORIES

9 g fat (4 g sat, 3 g mono)
46 mg cholesterol
7 g carbohydrate
27 g protein
2 g fiber
332 mg sodium
278 mg potassium

NUTRITION BONUS:
Zinc (27% daily value)
Iron (15% dv)

Healthy)(Weight

Lower ⬇ Carbs

ACTIVE TIME: **40 MINUTES**

TOTAL: **40 MINUTES**

TO MAKE AHEAD: **Prepare the steak roll (Steps 2-4). Wrap tightly in plastic wrap and refrigerate for up to 6 hours. When ready to grill, proceed with Steps 5 and 6.**

EQUIPMENT: **Meat mallet, skewers**

VARIATION:

■ Substitute ½ cup chopped roasted red peppers or ½ cup chopped artichoke hearts for the sun-dried tomatoes (skip Step 2). Mash ½ cup blue cheese with 2 tablespoons milk until smooth and substitute for the Boursin in Step 4.

ACTIVE TIME: **25 MINUTES**

TOTAL: **25 MINUTES**

INGREDIENT NOTE:

■ Shao Hsing (or Shaoxing) is a seasoned rice wine. It is available in most Asian specialty markets and some larger supermarkets in the Asian section. Dry sherry is an acceptable substitute.

SPICY BEEF WITH SHRIMP & BOK CHOY

Like fish sauce or anchovies, pungent oyster sauce mellows brilliantly in sauce, creating a salty back taste that works well with greens (here, bok choy) and especially with beef. If you want to forgo rice, try shredded jícama, carrots and zucchini as a bed for this easy supper.

¼	cup Shao Hsing rice wine (*see Note*)
1 ½	tablespoons oyster-flavored sauce
2	teaspoons cornstarch
4	teaspoons canola oil, divided
¾	pound sirloin steak, trimmed of fat, cut in half lengthwise and thinly sliced
¼ -½	teaspoon crushed red pepper
10	raw shrimp (21-25 per pound), peeled, deveined and chopped
1	pound bok choy, preferably baby bok choy, trimmed and sliced into 1-inch pieces

1. Whisk rice wine, oyster sauce and cornstarch in a small bowl until the cornstarch is dissolved.

2. Heat 2 teaspoons oil in a large nonstick skillet or wok over medium-high heat. Add beef and crushed red pepper; cook, stirring, until the beef begins to brown, 1 to 2 minutes. Add shrimp and continue to cook, stirring, until the shrimp is opaque and pink, 1 to 2 minutes. Transfer the beef, shrimp and any juices to a plate.

3. Heat the remaining 2 teaspoons oil over medium-high heat in the same pan. Add bok choy and cook, stirring, until it begins to wilt, 2 to 4 minutes. Stir in the cornstarch mixture. Return the beef-shrimp mixture to the pan and cook, stirring, until heated through and the sauce has thickened slightly, about 1 minute.

MAKES 4 SERVINGS, ABOUT 1 CUP EACH.

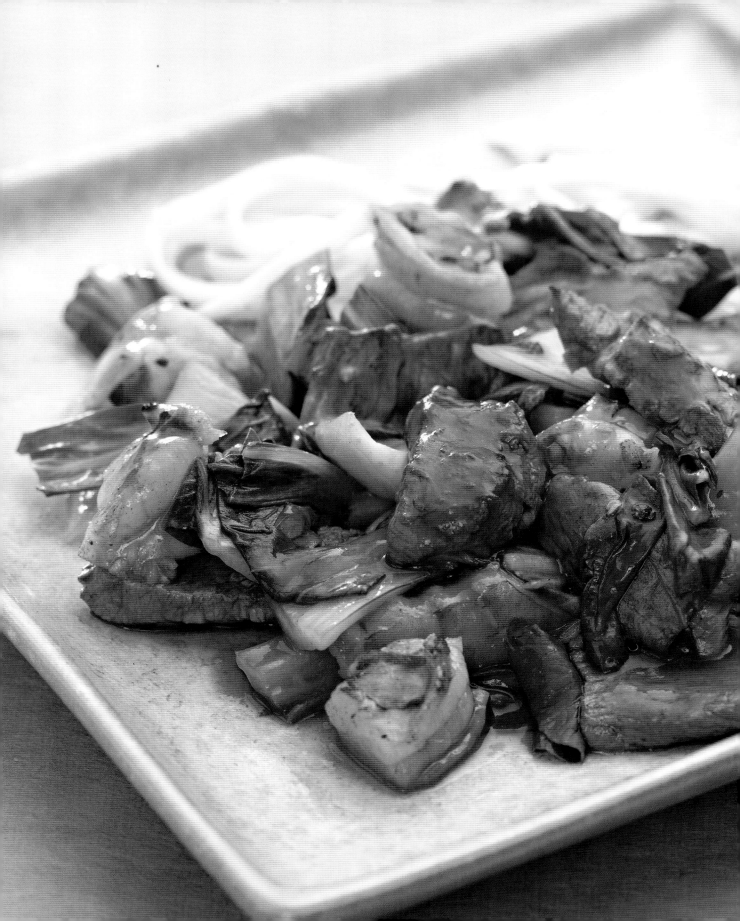

ACTIVE TIME: **1 HOUR**

TOTAL: **3¼ HOURS**

TO MAKE AHEAD: **The chili will keep, covered, in the refrigerator for up to 2 days or in the freezer for up to 2 months.**

VARIATION:

■ For a hot, smoky chili, add 1 tablespoon chopped chipotle pepper in adobo sauce.

ULTIMATE BEEF CHILI

Make this hearty chili even more satisfying and colorful by offering vegetable garnishes like chopped scallions and chopped fresh tomatoes. Serve it with warmed corn tortillas and a green salad topped with orange slices.

1	pound beef round, trimmed and cut into ½-inch chunks
	Salt & freshly ground pepper to taste
1½	tablespoons canola oil, divided
3	onions, chopped
1	green bell pepper, seeded and chopped
1	red bell pepper, seeded and chopped
6	cloves garlic, minced
2	jalapeño peppers, seeded and finely chopped
2	tablespoons ground cumin
2	tablespoons chili powder
1	tablespoon paprika
2	teaspoons dried oregano
12	ounces dark *or* light beer
1	28-ounce can diced tomatoes
8	sun-dried tomatoes (*not* packed in oil), snipped into small pieces
2	bay leaves
3	19-ounce cans dark kidney beans, rinsed
¼	cup chopped fresh cilantro
2	tablespoons lime juice

1. Season beef with salt and pepper. In a Dutch oven, heat ½ tablespoon oil over medium-high heat. Add half the beef and sauté until browned on all sides, 2 to 5 minutes. Transfer to a plate lined with paper towels. Repeat with another ½ tablespoon oil and remaining beef; set aside.

2. Reduce heat to medium and add remaining ½ tablespoon oil. Add onions and bell peppers; cook, stirring frequently, until onions are golden brown, 10 to 20 minutes. Add garlic, jalapeños, cumin, chili powder, paprika and oregano. Stir until aromatic, about 2 minutes.

3. Add beer and simmer, scraping up any browned bits, for about 3 minutes. Add diced tomatoes, sun-dried tomatoes, bay leaves and reserved beef. Cover and simmer, stirring occasionally, until beef is very tender, 1½ to 2 hours.

4. Add beans; cook, covered, stirring occasionally, until chili has thickened, 30 to 45 minutes. Remove bay leaves. Stir in cilantro and lime juice. Adjust seasoning with salt and pepper.

MAKES **12** SERVINGS, **1** CUP EACH.

PICADILLO

Picadillo, which means "small bits and pieces," is a sweet-and-savory spiced ground-meat mixture from Latin America. It's traditionally made with beef and pork, but using lean ground turkey breast instead cuts the saturated fat dramatically. Serve it with warm corn or whole-wheat flour tortillas

2	eggs (optional)
1	pound lean ground beef *or* ground turkey breast
2	teaspoons extra-virgin olive oil
1	medium onion, chopped
½	cup chopped scallions, divided
3	cloves garlic, minced
4	teaspoons chili powder
1 ½	teaspoons dried oregano
1 ½	teaspoons ground cumin
¾	teaspoon ground cinnamon
⅛	teaspoon cayenne pepper
½	cup golden raisins
½	cup chopped pitted green olives
2	tablespoons tomato paste
1	cup water
½	teaspoon freshly ground pepper

1. If using eggs, place in a small saucepan and cover with cold water. Bring to a boil; simmer on medium-low for 10 minutes. Drain; let cool; peel and slice.

2. Meanwhile, cook meat in a large nonstick skillet over medium-high heat, crumbling it with a wooden spoon, until no longer pink, about 5 minutes. Transfer to a colander; drain off fat.

3. Add oil to the skillet. Add onion, ¼ cup scallions and garlic; cook over medium heat, stirring often, until softened, 2 to 3 minutes. Stir in chili powder, oregano, cumin, cinnamon and cayenne; cook, stirring, until fragrant, about 1 minute. Add raisins, olives, tomato paste, water and the browned meat; stir to blend. Reduce heat to low, cover and simmer, stirring occasionally, for 10 minutes. Season with pepper. Garnish with the remaining scallions and the hard-boiled eggs, if desired.

MAKES 4 SERVINGS, 1 CUP EACH.

PER SERVING (WITH BEEF):

313 CALORIES

13 g fat (3 g sat, 7 g mono)

70 mg cholesterol

25 g carbohydrate

26 g protein

4 g fiber

558 mg sodium

754 mg potassium

NUTRITION BONUS:
Iron (25% daily value)
Vitamin A (20% dv)
Vitamin C (15% dv)

PER SERVING (WITH TURKEY):

277 CALORIES

9 g fat (0 g sat, 5 g mono)

45 mg cholesterol

25 g carbohydrate

30 g protein

4 g fiber

548 mg sodium

362 mg potassium

NUTRITION BONUS:
Vitamin A (20% daily value)
Iron (15% dv)
Vitamin C (15% dv)

Healthy ⚓ Weight

ACTIVE TIME: **30 MINUTES**

TOTAL: **40 MINUTES**

279 CALORIES

13 g fat (4 g sat, 6 g mono)

95 mg cholesterol

10 g carbohydrate

29 g protein

2 g fiber

487 mg sodium

523 mg potassium

NUTRITION BONUS:
Zinc (27% daily value)
Iron, Potassium &
Vitamin A (15% dv)

Healthy)(Weight

Lower ⬇ Carbs

ACTIVE TIME: **1 HOUR**

TOTAL: **5-6 HOURS**

TO MAKE AHEAD: **Cover and refrigerate for up to 3 days or freeze for up to 2 months.**

INGREDIENT NOTES:

- Levels of sodium in tomato paste vary from 20 mg to 290 mg per 2 tablespoons. To find the lower-sodium varieties, check the label.

- Boston butt (or "Boston-style butt," "fresh pork butt," "pork shoulder") can weigh upwards of 10 pounds, so you may have to ask your butcher to cut one down.

PULLED PORK

This is slow cooking at its best: pork cooked to fall-apart tenderness in a deeply flavored, spicy-sweet sauce. Serve it up on whole-wheat buns at your next tailgate party, and pass around plenty of napkins!

1	tablespoon extra-virgin olive oil
2	medium yellow onions, diced
2	tablespoons chili powder
1	tablespoon cumin
2	teaspoons paprika
1	teaspoon cayenne
12	ounces beer, preferably lager (1 ½ cups)
¾	cup ketchup
¾	cup cider vinegar
½	cup whole-grain mustard
2	tablespoons tomato paste (*see Note*)
1	canned chipotle pepper in adobo sauce, minced, plus 1 tablespoon adobo sauce
1	5-pound bone-in Boston butt (*see Note*)

1. Preheat oven to 300°F. Heat oil in a large Dutch oven over medium-low heat. Add onions and cook, stirring occasionally, until lightly browned and very soft, about 20 minutes.

2. Increase heat to high; add chili powder, cumin, paprika and cayenne and cook, stirring, until fragrant, 1 minute. Add beer, ketchup, vinegar, mustard, tomato paste, chipotle pepper and adobo sauce; bring to a boil. Reduce heat to medium-low and simmer, uncovered, stirring occasionally, until the sauce is slightly thickened, 10 minutes. Meanwhile, trim all visible fat from the pork.

3. Remove the pan from the heat and add the pork, spooning sauce over it. Cover the pan, transfer to the oven and bake for 1½ hours. Turn the pork over, cover, and bake for 1½ hours more. Uncover and bake until a fork inserted into the meat turns easily, 1 to 2 hours more.

4. Transfer the pork to a large bowl and cover with foil. Pour the sauce into a large measuring cup or glass bowl and refrigerate until the fat and sauce begin to separate, 15 minutes. Skim off the fat. Return the sauce to the pan and heat over medium-high until hot, about 4 minutes.

5. Remove the bone and any remaining pieces of fat from the meat. The bone should easily slip away from the tender meat. Pull the pork apart into long shreds using two forks. Add the hot sauce to the meat; stir to combine. Serve hot.

MAKES **12** SERVINGS, **3** OUNCES EACH.

GRILLED PORK TENDERLOIN WITH MUSTARD, ROSEMARY & APPLE MARINADE

This recipe gets added depth and a pretty finish from a balsamic vinaigrette that's enriched with either port or black tea. Try the boldly flavored marinade with chicken too.

¼ cup frozen apple juice concentrate
2 tablespoons plus 1 ½ teaspoons Dijon mustard
2 tablespoons extra-virgin olive oil, divided
2 tablespoons chopped fresh rosemary *or* thyme
4 cloves garlic, minced
1 teaspoon crushed peppercorns
2 12-ounce pork tenderloins, trimmed of fat
1 tablespoon minced shallot
3 tablespoons port *or* brewed black tea
2 tablespoons balsamic vinegar
¼ teaspoon salt, or to taste
 Freshly ground pepper to taste

1. Whisk apple juice concentrate, 2 tablespoons mustard, 1 tablespoon oil, rosemary (or thyme), garlic and peppercorns in a small bowl. Reserve 3 tablespoons marinade for basting. Place tenderloins in a shallow glass dish and pour the remaining marinade over them, turning to coat. Cover and marinate in the refrigerator for at least 20 minutes or for up to 2 hours, turning several times.

2. Heat a grill or broiler.

3. Combine shallot, port (or tea), vinegar, salt, pepper and the remaining 1 ½ teaspoons mustard and 1 tablespoon oil in a small bowl or a jar with a tight-fitting lid; whisk or shake until blended. Set aside.

4. Remove the tenderloins from the marinade (discard used marinade). Grill or broil, turning several times and basting the browned sides with the reserved marinade until just cooked through, 15 to 20 minutes. (An instant-read thermometer inserted in the center should register 155°F. The temperature will increase to 160° during resting.)

5. Transfer the tenderloins to a clean cutting board, tent with foil and let rest for about 5 minutes before carving them into ½-inch-thick slices. Arrange the pork slices on plates and drizzle with the shallot dressing. Serve immediately.

MAKES 6 SERVINGS.

PER SERVING:

165 CALORIES

5 g fat (1 g sat, 2 g mono)
63 mg cholesterol
5 g carbohydrate
23 g protein
0 g fiber
186 mg sodium
397 mg potassium

NUTRITION BONUS:
Vitamin C (20% daily value)

Healthy ⟩⟨ Weight

Lower ⬇ Carbs

ACTIVE TIME: **20 MINUTES**

TOTAL: **1 HOUR**

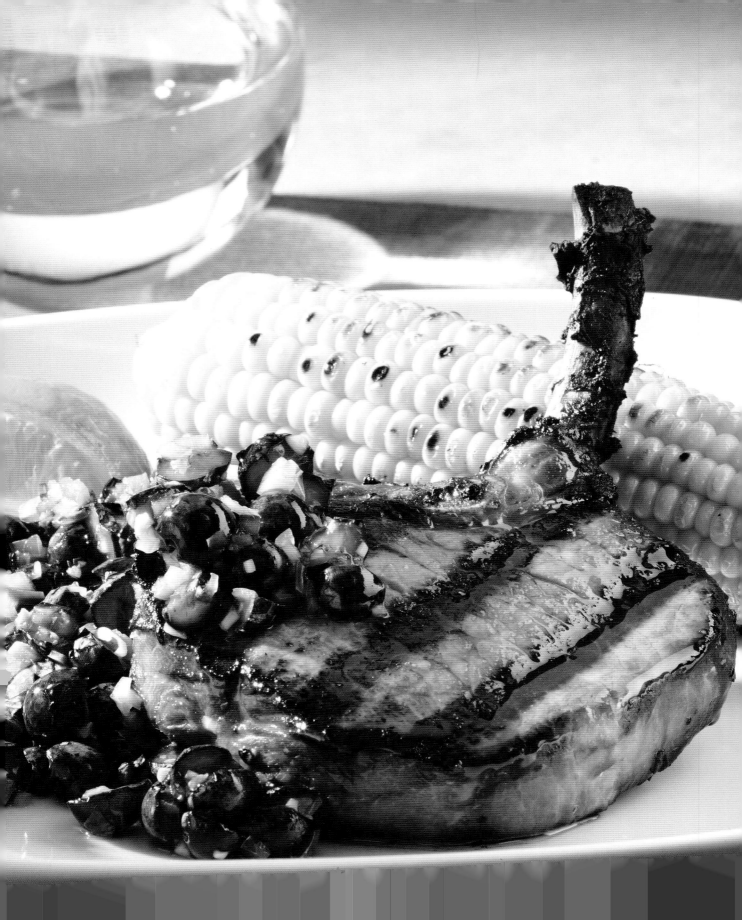

TERIYAKI PORK CHOPS WITH BLUEBERRY-GINGER RELISH

Take five minutes in the morning to get these pork chops marinating so they're ready to grill the same night or even the next day. Serve with grilled corn on the cob and a quick stir-fry of bok choy, broccoli and scallions.

4 bone-in center-cut pork chops (about 1 ¾ pounds), trimmed of fat

MARINADE

3 tablespoons reduced-sodium soy sauce
2 tablespoons dry sherry (*see Ingredient Note, page 245*)
2 cloves garlic, crushed
1 teaspoon brown sugar
¼ teaspoon crushed red pepper

BLUEBERRY-GINGER RELISH

1 cup fresh blueberries, coarsely chopped
1 shallot, chopped
1 serrano chile, seeded and minced
1 tablespoon chopped fresh cilantro
1 tablespoon lime juice
1 teaspoon minced fresh ginger
¼ teaspoon salt

1. To marinate: Place pork chops in a large sealable plastic bag. Whisk soy sauce, sherry, garlic, brown sugar and crushed red pepper in a small bowl. Add the marinade to the bag, seal and turn to coat. Marinate in the refrigerator for at least 2 hours or overnight.

2. To prepare relish: About 20 minutes before grilling the pork, combine blueberries, shallot, chile, cilantro, lime juice, ginger and salt in a small bowl.

3. Preheat grill to high. Remove the pork chops from the marinade (discard marinade). Grill the chops 3 to 5 minutes per side. Let them rest for 5 minutes before serving with the relish.

MAKES 4 SERVINGS, 1 CHOP & ¼ CUP RELISH EACH.

PER SERVING:

229 CALORIES

8 g fat (3 g sat, 4 g mono)
81 mg cholesterol
7 g carbohydrate
30 g protein
1 g fiber
273 mg sodium
440 mg potassium

NUTRITION BONUS:
Selenium (67% daily value)

Healthy ⚖ Weight

Lower ⬇ Carbs

ACTIVE TIME: **30 MINUTES**

TOTAL: **2½ HOURS**
(including 2 hours marinating time)

TO MAKE AHEAD: **Marinate the pork (Step 1) for up to 1 day.**

EASY SIDE DISHES

GRAINS & POTATOES
Asian Brown Rice

Cook 1 cup brown rice (*see page 228*), adding 2 teaspoons minced fresh ginger to 2½ cups cooking liquid. Stir 1 diced red bell pepper, ½ cup chopped water chestnuts and 1 teaspoon each reduced-sodium soy sauce and toasted sesame oil into the cooked rice. MAKES **6** SERVINGS.

PER SERVING: **127** calories; 2 g fat (0 g sat, 1 g mono); 0 mg cholesterol; 25 g carbohydrate; 3 g protein; 3 g fiber; 32 mg sodium; 123 mg potassium. NUTRITION BONUS: **Vitamin C (60% daily value).**

Brown Rice & Greens

Cook 1 cup brown rice (*see page 228*). Stir 2 cups baby spinach or arugula into the hot rice, cover and let stand for 5 minutes. Season with salt and freshly ground pepper. MAKES **6** SERVINGS.

PER SERVING: **113** calories; 1 g fat (0 g sat, 0 g mono); 0 mg cholesterol; 24 g carbohydrate; 2 g protein; 2 g fiber; 111 mg sodium; 77 mg potassium.

Buttermilk-Herb Mashed Potatoes

Peel 2 large Yukon Gold potatoes and cut into chunks. Place in a medium saucepan and cover with water. Add 2 peeled garlic cloves. Bring to a boil; cook until the potatoes are tender. Drain; add 2 teaspoons butter and ¼ cup nonfat buttermilk, and mash with a potato masher to the desired consistency. Stir in 1 tablespoon chopped fresh herbs. Season with salt and freshly ground pepper. MAKES **4** SERVINGS.

PER SERVING: **85** calories; 2 g fat (1 g sat, 0 g mono); 5 mg cholesterol; 14 g carbohydrate; 2 g protein; 1 g fiber; 87 mg sodium; 416 mg potassium.

Garlic-Tomato Toasts

Grill or toast 4 slices whole-wheat country bread. Cut 2 garlic cloves in half. Rub the tops of the bread with the cut sides of the garlic and drizzle with 2 teaspoons extra-virgin olive oil. Cut 2 plum tomatoes in half and rub the toasts with the cut sides of the tomato halves. Sprinkle with kosher salt and coarsely ground pepper. MAKES **4** SERVINGS.

PER SERVING: **91** calories; 4 g fat (1 g sat, 2 g mono); 0 mg cholesterol; 13 g carbohydrate; 3 g protein; 2 g fiber; 183 mg sodium; 82 mg potassium. NUTRITION BONUS: **Selenium (15% daily value).**

Oven Fries

Preheat oven to 450°F. Cut 2 large Yukon Gold potatoes into wedges. Toss with 4 teaspoons extra-virgin olive oil, ½ teaspoon salt and ½ teaspoon dried thyme (optional). Spread the wedges out on a rimmed baking sheet. Bake until browned and tender, turning once, about 20 minutes total. MAKES **4** SERVINGS.

PER SERVING: **103** calories; 5 g fat (1 g sat, 4 g mono); 0 mg cholesterol; 13 g carbohydrate; 2 g protein; 1 g fiber; 291 mg sodium; 407 mg potassium.

Oven Sweet Potato Fries

Preheat oven to 450°F. Peel 2 large sweet potatoes and cut into wedges. Toss with 4 teaspoons canola oil, ½ teaspoon salt and a pinch of cayenne. Spread the wedges out on a rimmed baking sheet. Bake until browned and tender, turning once, about 20 minutes total. MAKES **4** SERVINGS.

PER SERVING: **122** calories; 5 g fat (0 g sat, 3 g mono); 0 mg cholesterol; 19 g carbohydrate; 2 g protein; 3 g fiber; 323 mg sodium; 429 mg potassium. NUTRITION BONUS: **Vitamin A (350% daily value), Vitamin C (30% dv).**

Provençal Barley

Toss 2 cups cooked barley (*see page 228*) with 2 chopped plum tomatoes, 4 chopped pitted Kalamata olives and ½ teaspoon herbes de Provence. MAKES **4** SERVINGS, ABOUT ½ CUP EACH.

PER SERVING: **115** calories; 1 g fat (0 g sat, 1 g mono); 0 mg cholesterol; 24 g carbohydrate; 2 g protein; 4 g fiber; 65 mg sodium; 157 mg potassium.

VEGETABLES
Asparagus with Fresh Tomato Sauce

Steam 1 pound asparagus. Combine 2 chopped tomatoes, 1 minced shallot, 1 tablespoon each extra-virgin olive oil and balsamic vinegar; season with salt and pepper. Top the asparagus with the tomato sauce.
MAKES 4 SERVINGS.
PER SERVING: 58 calories; 4 g fat (1 g sat, 3 g mono); 0 mg cholesterol; 5 g carbohydrate; 2 g protein; 2 g fiber; 85 mg sodium; 274 mg potassium.
NUTRITION BONUS: Folate (23% daily value).

Lemon Lovers' Asparagus

Preheat oven to 450°F. Trim 2 bunches of asparagus and thinly slice 2 lemons. Toss on a rimmed baking sheet with 2 tablespoons extra-virgin olive oil, 4 teaspoons chopped fresh oregano and ½ teaspoon each salt and freshly ground pepper. Roast, shaking the pan occasionally, until tender-crisp, 10 to 15 minutes.
MAKES 4 SERVINGS.
PER SERVING: 91 calories; 7 g fat (1 g sat, 5 g mono); 0 mg cholesterol; 9 g carbohydrate; 2 g protein; 4 g fiber; 302 mg sodium; 241 mg potassium.
NUTRITION BONUS: Vitamin C (80% daily value), Folate (27% dv), Vitamin A (15% dv).

Mary's Zucchini with Parmesan

Slice 2 pounds zucchini ¼ inch thick. Cook with 2 teaspoons extra-virgin olive oil in a large nonstick skillet, stirring every 2 to 3 minutes, until tender and golden. Reduce heat; season with salt and freshly ground pepper to taste. Sprinkle with ½ cup finely grated Parmesan cheese, cover and cook until the cheese is melted.
MAKES 4 SERVINGS, ¾ CUP EACH.
PER SERVING: 83 calories; 5 g fat (1 g sat, 2 g mono); 5 mg cholesterol; 8 g carbohydrate; 5 g protein; 3 g fiber; 277 mg sodium; 594 mg potassium.
NUTRITION BONUS: Vitamin C (60% daily value).

Sautéed Watercress

Sauté 2 minced garlic cloves in 4 teaspoons extra-virgin olive oil in a large nonstick skillet until fragrant. Add 1 pound watercress (tough stems removed). Cook, stirring often, until wilted. Stir in a splash of champagne (or white-wine) vinegar and season to taste with salt and freshly ground pepper.
MAKES 4 SERVINGS, ABOUT ½ CUP EACH.
PER SERVING: 56 calories; 5 g fat (1 g sat, 4 g mono); 0 mg cholesterol; 2 g carbohydrate; 3 g protein; 1 g fiber; 116 mg sodium; 350 mg potassium.
NUTRITION BONUS: Vitamin A (100% daily value), Vitamin C (80% dv), Calcium (15% dv).

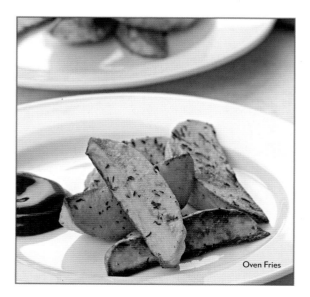
Oven Fries

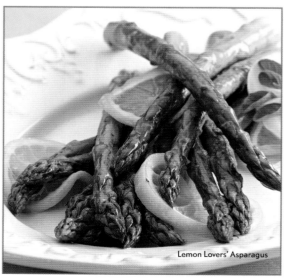
Lemon Lovers' Asparagus

Sesame Green Beans

Preheat oven to 500°F. Trim 1 pound green beans. Toss with 2 teaspoons extra-virgin olive oil. Spread in an even layer on a rimmed baking sheet. Roast, turning once halfway through cooking, until tender and beginning to brown, about 10 minutes. Toss with 2 teaspoons toasted sesame seeds, 1 teaspoon sesame oil, salt and freshly ground pepper to taste.
MAKES 4 SERVINGS.
PER SERVING: 67 calories; 4 g fat (1 g sat, 3 g mono); 0 mg cholesterol; 7 g carbohydrate; 2 g protein; 4 g fiber; 73 mg sodium; 280 mg potassium.
NUTRITION BONUS: Vitamin C (15% daily value).

Trio of Peas

Sauté 1 cup each trimmed snow peas and sugar snap peas in 2 teaspoons canola oil in a large nonstick skillet. Stir in 2 cups frozen peas and heat through. Remove from the heat; stir in ½ teaspoon freshly grated lemon zest, 4 teaspoons lemon juice, 1½ teaspoon dried tarragon, 1 teaspoon butter and a pinch of salt.
MAKES 6 SERVINGS, ABOUT ½ CUP EACH.
PER SERVING: 74 calories; 2 g fat (1 g sat, 1 g mono); 2 mg cholesterol; 10 g carbohydrate; 3 g protein; 4 g fiber; 84 mg sodium; 126 mg potassium.
NUTRITION BONUS: Vitamin C (30% daily value), Vitamin A (25% dv).

Vegetable Stir-Fry

Stir-fry a 16-ounce package of frozen stir-fry vegetables with 1 teaspoon peanut oil (or canola oil). Toss with 2 tablespoons oyster sauce (or hoisin sauce) and 1 tablespoon rice vinegar.
MAKES 4 SERVINGS.
PER SERVING: 53 calories; 1 g fat (0 g sat, 1 g mono); 0 mg cholesterol; 10 g carbohydrate; 3 g protein; 3 g fiber; 405 mg sodium; 213 mg potassium.
NUTRITION BONUS: Vitamin A (90% daily value), Vitamin C (40% dv).

Wilted Spinach with Garlic

Heat 1 tablespoon extra-virgin olive oil in a large skillet over medium-high heat. Add 1 minced garlic clove and cook, stirring, about 30 seconds. Add 1 pound stemmed spinach; cook, stirring, until just wilted, 2 to 4 minutes. Season with salt and freshly ground pepper.
MAKES 4 SERVINGS.
PER SERVING: 59 calories; 4 g fat (1 g sat, 3 g mono); 0 mg cholesterol; 4 g carbohydrate; 3 g protein; 3 g fiber; 162 mg sodium; 636 mg potassium.
NUTRITION BONUS: Vitamin A (210% daily value), Folate (55% dv), Vitamin C (50% dv), Magnesium (22% dv), Potassium (18% dv), Iron (15% dv).

Zesty Green Beans & Peppers

Preheat oven to 450°F. Toss 1 pound trimmed green beans and 1 thinly sliced red bell pepper with 1 tablespoon extra-virgin olive oil, zest of 1 orange, ½ teaspoon salt and ¼ teaspoon crushed red pepper. Roast on a rimmed baking sheet, turning once halfway through, until tender and slightly wilted, about 10 minutes.
MAKES 4 SERVINGS, ¾ CUP EACH.
PER SERVING: 78 calories; 4 g fat (1 g sat, 3 g mono); 0 mg cholesterol; 11 g carbohydrate; 2 g protein; 5 g fiber; 298 mg sodium; 318 mg potassium.
NUTRITION BONUS: Vitamin C (150% daily value), Vitamin A (40% dv).

Zucchini & Mushroom Sauté

Julienne 2 small zucchini. Sauté with 2 teaspoons extra-virgin olive oil in a large nonstick skillet over high heat for 2 minutes. Add 1½ cups sliced mushrooms and 2 teaspoons chopped fresh basil and sauté until softened, about 1 minute. Season with salt and freshly ground pepper.
MAKES 4 SERVINGS.
PER SERVING: 37 calories; 4 g fat (0 g sat, 2 g mono); 0 mg cholesterol; 3 g carbohydrate; 2 g protein; 1 g fiber; 80 mg sodium; 240 mg potassium.
NUTRITION BONUS: Vitamin C (20% daily value).

VEGETABLE-COOKING GUIDE

Start with 1 pound untrimmed raw vegetables for 4 servings. (*For calorie information, see page 240.*)

Artichokes, Baby

Look for: Tight, small heads, no browning or bruising.
Prep: Snip off tough outer leaves; cut off top quarter and trim off woody stem.
Grill: Halve artichokes, scoop out the choke if necessary, then toss with 1 tablespoon extra-virgin olive oil and ½ teaspoon kosher salt. Preheat grill. Place the artichokes over direct, medium-high heat and cook, turning once or twice, until tender, about 8 minutes.
Microwave: Place artichokes in a large glass baking dish, add ½ cup white wine (or dry vermouth), ½ teaspoon salt and 1 teaspoon dried thyme. Cover tightly and microwave on High until tender, about 8 minutes.
Steam: Place artichokes in a steamer basket over 1 inch of water in a large pot set over high heat. Cover and steam until tender, about 15 minutes.

Asparagus

Look for: Sturdy spears with tight heads; cut ends not desiccated or woody. Fresh asparagus snaps when bent.
Prep: Trim off stem ends; shave down any woody bits with a vegetable peeler.
Braise: Place a large skillet over high heat. Add asparagus, ½ cup water and a slice of lemon. Cover, bring to a simmer, and cook until tender, about 5 minutes.
Grill: Preheat grill; lightly oil rack. Place asparagus over direct, medium heat; cook until browned, turning occasionally, about 6 minutes.
Microwave: Place asparagus in a large glass baking dish; add ¼ cup water, drizzle with 1 teaspoon extra-virgin olive oil, and cover tightly. Microwave on High until tender, about 3 minutes.
Roast: Preheat oven to 500°F. Spread asparagus on a baking sheet or in a pan large enough to hold it in a single layer. Coat with 2 teaspoons extra-virgin olive oil. Roast, turning once halfway through cooking, until wilted and browned, about 10 minutes.

Beets

Look for: Small; firm, richly colored.
Prep: Peel.
Microwave: Cut beets into ¼-inch-thick rings; place in a large glass baking dish. Add ¼ cup water, cover tightly and microwave on High for 10 minutes. Let stand, covered, for 5 minutes before serving.
Roast: Preheat oven to 500°F. Cut beets into 1½-inch chunks. Spread on a baking sheet or in a pan large enough to hold them in a single layer. Coat with 2 teaspoons extra-virgin olive oil. Roast, turning once halfway through cooking, until tender, about 30 minutes.
Steam: Cut beets into quarters. Place in a steamer basket over 1 inch of water in a large pot set over high heat. Cover and steam until tender, about 15 minutes.

Broccoli

Look for: Sturdy, dark-green spears with tight buds, no yellowing and a high floret-to-stem ratio.
Prep: Cut off florets; cut stalks in half lengthwise and then into 1-inch-thick half-moons.
Microwave: Place stems and florets in a large glass baking dish. Cover tightly and microwave on High until tender, about 4 minutes.
Roast: Preheat oven to 500°F. Spread on a baking sheet or in a pan large enough to hold them in a single layer. Coat with 1 tablespoon extra-virgin olive oil. Roast, turning once halfway through cooking, until tender and browned in places, about 10 minutes.
Steam: Place stems in a steamer basket over 1 inch of water (with 1 tablespoon lemon juice added to it) in a large pot set over high heat. Cover and steam for 2 minutes. Add florets; cover and continue steaming until tender, about 5 minutes more.

Carrots

Look for: Orange, firm; no gray, white or desiccated residue on skin; greens preferably still attached.
Prep: Peel; cut off greens.
Microwave: Cut carrots into ⅛-inch-thick rounds. Place in a large glass baking dish. Add ¼ cup broth (or white wine). Cover tightly and microwave on High until tender, about 3 minutes.
Roast: Preheat oven to 500°F. Cut carrots in half lengthwise then slice into 1½-inch-long pieces. Spread on a baking sheet or in a pan large enough to hold them in a single layer. Coat with 2 teaspoons extra-virgin olive oil. Roast, turning once halfway through cooking, until beginning to brown, about 15 minutes.
Sauté: Cut carrots into ⅛-inch-thick rounds. Melt 1 tablespoon butter in a large skillet over medium-low heat. Add carrots; stir and cook until tender, about 4 minutes. Add 1 teaspoon sugar; stir until glazed.
Steam: Cut carrots into ⅛-inch thick rounds. Place in a steamer basket over 1 inch of water in a large pot set over high heat. Cover and steam for 4 minutes.

Cauliflower

Look for: Tight white or purple heads without brown or yellow spots; the green leaves at the stem should still be attached firmly to the head, not limp or withered.

Prep: Cut into 1-inch-wide florets; discard core and thick stems.

Microwave: Place florets in a large glass baking dish. Add ¼ cup dry white wine (or dry vermouth). Cover tightly and microwave on High until tender, about 4 minutes.

Roast: Preheat oven to 500°F. Spread florets on a baking sheet or in a pan large enough to hold them in a single layer. Coat with 1 tablespoon extra-virgin olive oil. Roast, turning once halfway through cooking, until tender and beginning to brown, about 15 minutes.

Steam: Place florets in a steamer basket over 1 inch of water in a large pot set over high heat. Cover and steam for 5 minutes.

Corn

Look for: Pale to dark green husks with moist silks; ears should feel heavy, the cob filling the husk well.

Grill: Pull back the husks without removing them; pull out the silks. Replace the husks; soak the ears in water for 20 minutes. Preheat grill. Place corn (in husks) over high heat and grill, turning occasionally, until lightly browned, about 5 minutes. Remove husks before serving.

Microwave: Husk corn and cut ears in thirds; place in a large glass baking dish. Cover tightly and microwave on High until tender, about 4 minutes.

Sauté: Remove kernels from cobs. Melt 2 teaspoons butter in a large skillet over medium heat. Add corn kernels; cook, stirring constantly, until tender, about 3 minutes. Stir in ½ teaspoon white-wine vinegar before serving.

Steam: Husk corn, then break or cut ears in half to fit in a steamer basket. Set over 1 inch of water in a large pot over high heat. Cover and steam until tender, about 4 minutes.

Eggplant

Look for: Smooth, glossy skins without wrinkles or spongy spots; each should feel heavy for its size.

Prep: Slice into ½-inch-thick rounds (peeling is optional).

Grill: Preheat grill. Brush eggplant slices lightly with extra-virgin olive oil. Place over medium-high heat and grill, turning once, until browned, about 8 minutes.

Roast: Preheat oven to 500°F. Brush both sides of eggplant slices with 2 teaspoons extra-virgin olive oil and arrange on a baking sheet or pan large enough to hold them in a single layer. Roast, turning once halfway through cooking, until tender, about 15 minutes.

Green Beans

Look for: Small, thin, firm beans.

Prep: Snip off stem ends.

Microwave: Place beans in a large glass baking dish. Add ¼ cup broth (or water). Cover tightly and microwave on High for 4 minutes.

Roast: Preheat oven to 500°F. Spread beans on a baking sheet or in a pan large enough to hold them in a single layer. Coat with 1 tablespoon extra-virgin olive oil. Roast, turning once halfway through cooking, until tender and beginning to brown, about 10 minutes.

Sauté: Heat 2 teaspoons walnut oil in a large skillet. Add beans; cook, stirring constantly, for 2 minutes.

Steam: Place beans in a steamer basket over 1 inch of water in a large pot set over high heat. Cover and steam for 5 minutes.

Peas

Look for: If fresh, look for firm, vibrant green pods without blotches and with the stem end still attached.

Prep: If fresh, zip open the hull, using the stem end as a tab. If frozen, do not defrost before using.

Microwave: Place peas in a large glass baking dish; add 2 tablespoons broth (or unsweetened apple juice). Cover tightly and microwave on High for 2 minutes.

Sauté: Heat 2 teaspoons butter in a large skillet over medium heat. Add peas; cook, stirring often, until bright green, about 3 minutes.

Steam: Place peas in a steamer basket over 1 inch of water in a large pot set over high heat. Cover and steam for 2 minutes.

Potatoes, Red or Yukon Gold

Look for: Small potatoes with firm skins that are not loose, papery or bruised.

Prep: Scrub off any dirt (peeling is optional; the skin is fiber-rich and the nutrients are clustered about ½ inch below the skin).

Roast: Preheat oven to 500°F. Halve potatoes then cut into ½-inch wedges. Spread on a baking sheet or in a pan large enough to hold them in a single layer. Coat with 2 teaspoons extra-virgin olive oil. Roast, stirring once halfway through cooking, until crispy and browned on the outside and tender on the inside, 20 to 25 minutes.

Steam: Place potatoes in a steamer basket over 2 inches of water in a large pot set over high heat. Cover and steam until tender when pierced with a fork, about 10 minutes.

Spinach & Swiss Chard

Look for: Supple, deeply colored leaves without mushy spots.

Prep: Rinse thoroughly to remove sand; remove thick stems and shred leaves into 2-inch pieces. Rinse leaves again but do not dry.

Braise: Heat 2 teaspoons walnut oil (or canola oil) in a large skillet over medium heat. Add spinach or chard and toss until wilted. Add ½ cup dry white wine or dry vermouth. Cover, reduce heat and cook, about 5 minutes. Uncover and cook until liquid is reduced to a glaze. Sprinkle 2 teaspoons balsamic vinegar (or rice vinegar) over the greens.

Squash, Acorn

Look for: Green, orange or white varietals with firm, smooth skins and no spongy spots.

Prep: Cut in quarters and scoop out the seeds.

Braise: Place squash in a pot with 2 cups unsweetened apple juice. Set over medium-high heat and bring to a simmer. Cover, reduce heat and cook until tender when pierced with a fork, about 20 minutes.

Microwave: Place squash in a large glass baking dish; add ½ cup water. Cover tightly and microwave on High for 15 minutes; let stand, covered, for 10 minutes.

Squash, Delicata

Look for: Small, firm squash with bright yellow or orange skins that have green veins branching like lightning through them.

Prep: Cut squash in half lengthwise, scoop out seeds and slice into thin half-moons (peeling is optional).

Microwave: Place squash in a large glass baking dish with ¼ cup broth (or water). Cover tightly and microwave on High for 10 minutes.

Sauté: Melt 2 teaspoons butter in a large skillet over medium heat. Add squash slices; cook, stirring frequently, until tender, about 10 minutes. Stir in a pinch of grated nutmeg before serving.

Steam: Place squash slices in a steamer basket over 1 inch of water in a large pot set over high heat. Cover and cook until tender, about 6 minutes.

Squash, Summer & Zucchini

Look for: No breaks, gashes or soft spots; smaller squash (under 8 inches) are sweeter and have fewer seeds.

Prep: Do not peel, but scrub off dirt; cut off stem ends.

Grill: Cut squash lengthwise into ¼-inch strips. Preheat grill; brush strips lightly with 1 tablespoon extra-virgin olive oil. Place over direct, medium heat; grill, turning once, until marked and lightly browned, 3 to 4 minutes.

Roast: Preheat oven to 500°F. Cut squash lengthwise into ¼-inch-thick slices. Spread on a baking sheet or in a pan large enough to hold them in a single layer. Coat with 2 teaspoons extra-virgin olive oil. Roast, turning once halfway through cooking, until tender, about 10 minutes.

Sauté: Cut squash into ¼-inch-thick rings. Heat 1 tablespoon extra-virgin olive oil in a large skillet over medium heat. Add 1 minced garlic clove and squash; cook, stirring frequently, until tender, about 7 minutes.

Steam: Cut squash into ½-inch-thick rings. Place in a steamer basket with a small onion, thinly sliced. Place over 1 inch of water in a large pot set over high heat. Cook until tender, about 5 minutes.

Sweet Potatoes

Look for: Taut if papery skins with tapered ends.

Prep: Scrub.

Braise: Peel sweet potatoes and cut into 1-inch pieces. Place in a large skillet with 1 cup vegetable broth, 1 teaspoon honey and ½ teaspoon dried thyme. Bring to a simmer over high heat; reduce heat, cover and cook until almost tender, about 15 minutes. Uncover, increase heat and cook until the liquid is reduced to a glaze, about 2 minutes.

Microwaving: Place sweet potatoes in a large glass baking dish; pierce with a knife. Microwave on High until soft, 8 to 12 minutes. Let stand for 5 minutes.

Roast: Preheat oven to 500°F. Halve sweet potatoes, then slice into ½-inch wedges. Spread on a baking sheet or in a pan large enough to hold them in a single layer. Coat with 2 teaspoons extra-virgin olive oil. Roast, turning once halfway through cooking, until browned and tender, 20 to 25 minutes.

GRAIN-COOKING GUIDE

Start with 1 cup uncooked grain; serving size is ½ cup cooked. (*For calorie information, see page 240.*)

	LIQUID (water/broth)	YIELD	DIRECTIONS
BARLEY Quick-cooking	1¾ cups	2 cups	Bring liquid to a boil; add barley. Reduce heat to low and simmer, covered, 10-12 minutes.
Pearl	2½ cups	3-3½ cups	Bring barley and liquid to a boil. Reduce heat to low and simmer, covered, 35-50 minutes.
BULGUR	1½ cups	2½-3 cups	Bring bulgur and liquid to a boil. Reduce heat to low; simmer, covered, until tender and most of the liquid has been absorbed, 10-15 minutes.
COUSCOUS Whole-wheat	1¾ cups	3-3½ cups	Bring liquid to a boil; stir in couscous. Remove from heat and let stand, covered, 5 minutes. Fluff with a fork.
QUINOA	2 cups	3 cups	Rinse in several changes of cold water. Bring quinoa and liquid to a boil. Reduce heat to low and simmer, covered, until tender and most of the liquid has been absorbed, 15-20 minutes. Fluff with a fork.
RICE Brown	2½ cups	3 cups	Bring rice and liquid to a boil. Reduce heat to low and simmer, covered, until tender and most of the liquid has been absorbed, 40-50 minutes. Let stand 5 minutes, then fluff with a fork.
Wild	At least 4 cups	2-2½ cups	Cook rice in a large saucepan of lightly salted boiling water until tender, 45-55 minutes. Drain.

IN A HURRY?: Make instant brown rice or instant wild rice, ready in under 10 minutes (follow the package instructions).

EASY SNACKS

Avocado Tea Sandwich

Flavor 1 tablespoon reduced-fat mayonnaise with ½ teaspoon lemon juice and ⅛ teaspoon cracked black pepper. Thinly spread on 8 very thin slices wheat bread and top with 2 ounces sliced smoked salmon, 1 sliced avocado and 12 cucumber slices.

MAKES 4 SANDWICHES.

PER SERVING: 143 calories; 6 g fat (4 g sat, 3 g mono); 3 mg cholesterol; 17 g carbohydrate; 6 g protein; 4 g fiber; 303 mg sodium; 129 mg potassium.

Butter-Bean Spread & Rice Cakes

Spread 2 tablespoons Butter-Bean Spread (*page 147*) on 1 brown rice cake.

MAKES 1 SERVING.

PER SERVING: 60 calories; 1 g fat (0 g sat, 1 g mono); 1 mg cholesterol; 11 g carbohydrate; 2 g protein; 1 g fiber; 97 mg sodium; 100 mg potassium.

Cajun Spiced Hard-Boiled Egg

Sprinkle 1 hard-boiled egg with ⅛ teaspoon Cajun spice blend.

MAKES 1 SERVING.

PER SERVING: 68 calories; 5 g fat (1 g sat, 2 g mono); 187 mg cholesterol; 0 g carbohydrate; 6 g protein; 0 g fiber; 122 mg sodium; 55 mg potassium.

Cereal Mix

Combine ¼ cup Cheerios, 1 tablespoon raisins, 1 tablespoon toasted pepitas and 1 tablespoon semisweet mini chocolate chips.

MAKES 1 SERVING.

PER SERVING: 124 calories; 5 g fat (2 g sat, 1 g mono); 0 mg cholesterol; 22 g carbohydrate; 2 g protein; 2 g fiber; 79 mg sodium; 196 mg potassium.

Cheesy Popcorn

Toss 4 cups hot popcorn with ½ cup freshly grated Parmesan and cayenne pepper to taste.

MAKES 4 SERVINGS, ABOUT 1 CUP EACH.

PER SERVING: 75 calories; 3 g fat (2 g sat, 1 g mono); 9 mg cholesterol; 7 g carbohydrate; 5 g protein; 1 g fiber; 154 mg sodium; 43 mg potassium.

Cucumbers & Cottage Cheese

Sprinkle ½ cup low-fat cottage cheese with ¼ teaspoon spice blend, such as Jane's Krazy Mixed-Up Salt. Cut ½ cucumber into spears and dip into cottage cheese.

MAKES 1 SERVING.

PER SERVING: 104 calories; 1 g fat (1 g sat, 0 g mono); 5 mg cholesterol; 9 g carbohydrate; 15 g protein; 1 g fiber; 599 mg sodium; 318 mg potassium.

Egg & Crispbread

Mix 1 chopped hard-boiled egg with 1 tablespoon dill pickle relish and 2 teaspoons reduced-fat mayonnaise. Spread egg mixture on 1 whole-grain crispbread cracker, such as Wasa.

MAKES 1 SERVING.

PER SERVING: 112 calories; 5 g fat (2 g sat, 2 g mono); 187 mg cholesterol; 10 g carbohydrate; 6 g protein; 1 g fiber; 217 mg sodium; 76 mg potassium.

Eggcetera

Dip slices of 4 hard-boiled eggs in 1 teaspoon extra-virgin olive oil. Sprinkle the eggs with ½ teaspoon each kosher salt and paprika.

MAKES 4 SERVINGS.

PER EGG: 88 calories; 6 g fat (2 g sat, 3 g mono); 212 mg cholesterol; 1 g carbohydrate; 6 g protein; 0 g fiber; 357 mg sodium; 63 mg potassium.

Gorp

Combine ½ ounce whole unpeeled almonds, ¼ ounce each unsalted dry-roasted peanuts and dried cranberries and 1 tablespoon chopped pitted dates. Toss in 1½ teaspoons chocolate chips for a treat.

MAKES 2 SERVINGS.

PER SERVING: 102 calories; 6 g fat (1 g sat, 3 g mono); 0 mg cholesterol; 11 g carbohydrate; 3 g protein; 2 g fiber; 29 mg sodium; 69 mg potassium.

Guacamole-Stuffed Eggs

Halve 6 hard-boiled eggs and remove the yolks. Fill each half with 2 teaspoons prepared guacamole. Sprinkle with cracked black pepper and kosher salt.
MAKES 6 SERVINGS.
PER SERVING: 55 calories; 3 g fat (1 g sat, 0 g mono); 0 mg cholesterol; 2 g carbohydrate; 4 g protein; 1 g fiber; 223 mg sodium; 48 mg potassium.

Ham & Pepper Roll-Ups

Spread 1 tablespoon reduced-fat cream cheese on 2 slices reduced-sodium deli ham, top with ½ cup red bell pepper slices and roll.
MAKES 1 SERVING.
PER SERVING: 100 calories; 5 g fat (2 g sat, 2 g mono); 24 mg cholesterol; 6 g carbohydrate; 8 g protein; 1 g fiber; 317 mg sodium; 284 mg potassium.

Hummus & Vegetables

Dip ¾ cup mixed vegetables, such as baby carrots, cherry tomatoes and red bell pepper slices, into 3 tablespoons prepared hummus.
MAKES 1 SERVING.
PER SERVING: 108 calories; 5 g fat (1 g sat, 2 g mono); 0 mg cholesterol; 13 g carbohydrate; 5 g protein; 5 g fiber; 195 mg sodium; 274 mg potassium.

Pears & Blue Cheese

Top 1 cup sliced water-packed canned pears with 1 tablespoon crumbled blue cheese.
MAKES 1 SERVING.
PER SERVING: 96 calories; 2 g fat (1 g sat, 1 g mono); 5 mg cholesterol; 19 g carbohydrate; 2 g protein; 4 g fiber; 104 mg sodium; 147 mg potassium.

The Perfect Snack

Combine ⅛ cup (¾ ounce) cubed part-skim Swiss cheese, ⅛ cup (½ ounce) cubed smoked turkey and ½ apple, cubed.
MAKES 1 SERVING.
PER SERVING: 123 calories; 2 g fat (1 g sat, 0 g mono); 13 mg cholesterol; 20 g carbohydrate; 9 g protein; 3 g fiber; 190 mg sodium; 171 mg potassium.

Pickled Beets & Cheese

Top ½ cup sliced prepared pickled beets with 1 tablespoon crumbled goat cheese or 1 tablespoon crumbled blue cheese.
MAKES 1 SERVING.
PER SERVING: 85 calories; 3 g fat (2 g sat, 1 g mono); 7 mg cholesterol; 13 g carbohydrate; 3 g protein; 1 g fiber; 78 mg sodium; 208 mg potassium.

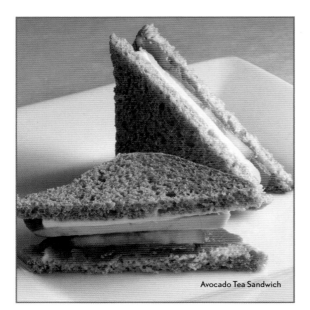
Avocado Tea Sandwich

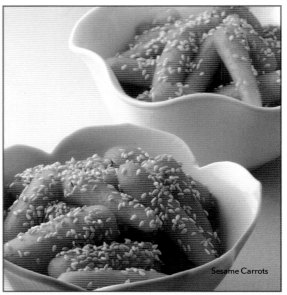
Sesame Carrots

Quick Kebabs

Thread ½ ounce each of cubed roasted deli turkey and Cheddar cheese, ¼ cup grapes and 6 dried apricots onto a wooden skewer.

MAKES 1 SERVING.

PER SERVING: 218 calories; 5 g fat (3 g sat, 1 g mono); 20 mg cholesterol; 37 g carbohydrate; 7 g protein; 5 g fiber; 247 mg sodium; 714 mg potassium.

Radish Crispbread

Spread 4 teaspoons reduced-fat chive cream cheese on 2 whole-grain crispbread crackers, such as Wasa, and top with ½ cup sliced radish *or* ½ cup sliced cucumber.

MAKES 1 SERVING.

PER SERVING: 104 calories; 4 g fat (2 g sat, 1 g mono); 11 mg cholesterol; 14 g carbohydrate; 4 g protein; 1 g fiber; 82 mg sodium; 183 mg potassium.

Sesame Carrots

Toss 2 cups of baby carrots with 1 tablespoon toasted sesame seeds and a pinch each of dried thyme and kosher salt.

MAKES 3 SERVINGS, ABOUT ⅔ CUP EACH.

PER SERVING: 33 calories; 0 g fat (0 g sat, 0 g mono); 0 mg cholesterol; 8 g carbohydrate; 1 g protein; 2 g fiber; 72 mg sodium; 220 mg potassium.

Shrimp Cocktail

Dip 4 large (21-25 per pound) shrimp in 2 tablespoons prepared cocktail sauce.

MAKES 1 SERVING.

PER SERVING: 74 calories; 1 g fat (0 g sat, 0 g mono); 86 mg cholesterol; 7 g carbohydrate; 10 g protein; 1 g fiber; 499 mg sodium; 215 mg potassium.

Sorbet Shake

Puree ½ cup each nonfat milk and fruit sorbet in a blender until combined. With the motor running, add 3 ice cubes and blend until smooth and thick.

MAKES 1 SERVING.

PER SERVING: 172 calories; 0 g fat (0 g sat, 0 g mono); 2 mg cholesterol; 39 g carbohydrate; 4 g protein; 1 g fiber; 51 mg sodium; 191 mg potassium.

Turkey Roll-Ups

Spread slices of deli turkey breast with honey mustard or mango chutney and season with freshly ground pepper. Wrap turkey around breadsticks. For a snappy touch, tie with a blanched chive.

MAKES 2 SERVINGS, 2 ROLL-UPS EACH.

PER SERVING: 82 calories; 4 g fat (1 g sat, 1 g mono); 10 mg cholesterol; 10 g carbohydrate; 3 g protein; 0 g fiber; 238 mg sodium; 47 mg potassium.

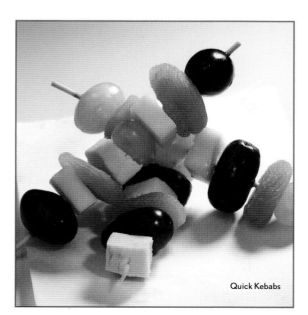

Quick Kebabs

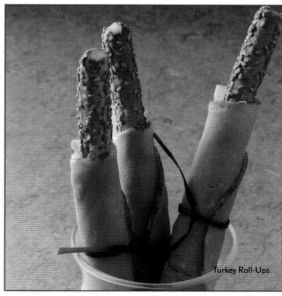

Turkey Roll-Ups

EASY DESSERTS

Balsamic-Spiked Strawberries

Wash and dry 1 pint strawberries. Hull and slice berries, place in a bowl and toss with 1 to 2 tablespoons sugar. Sprinkle with 2 to 3 teaspoons balsamic vinegar. Let stand for 20 minutes.

MAKES 4 SERVINGS.

PER SERVING: 40 calories; 0 g fat (0 g sat, 0 g mono); 0 mg cholesterol; 10 g carbohydrate; 1 g protein; 2 g fiber; 1 mg sodium; 112 mg potassium.

Banana-Cinnamon Frozen Yogurt

Soften 1 pint nonfat vanilla frozen yogurt. Mash together 2 small bananas, 1 teaspoon lemon juice and ½ teaspoon ground cinnamon. Add the frozen yogurt and mix well with a whisk. Scoop into 4 dessert dishes, cover and freeze until firm, about 30 minutes.

MAKES 4 SERVINGS.

PER SERVING: 126 calories; 0 g fat (0 g sat, 0 g mono); 0 mg cholesterol; 30 g carbohydrate; 4 g protein; 1 g fiber; 41 mg sodium; 304 mg potassium.

Broiled Mango

Preheat broiler. Position rack in upper third of oven. Peel and slice 1 mango. Arrange mango slices in a single layer in a broiler pan covered with foil. Broil until browned in spots, 8 to 10 minutes. Squeeze lime juice over the broiled mango and serve.

MAKES 2 SERVINGS.

PER SERVING: 69 calories; 0 g fat (0 g sat, 0 g mono); 0 mg cholesterol; 18 g carbohydrate; 1 g protein; 2 g fiber; 2 mg sodium; 167 mg potassium.

Cherries with Ricotta & Toasted Almonds

Heat ¾ cup frozen pitted cherries in the microwave. Top cherries with 2 tablespoons part-skim ricotta and 1 tablespoon toasted slivered almonds.

MAKES 1 SERVING.

PER SERVING: 150 calories; 6 g fat (2 g sat, 3 g mono); 10 mg cholesterol; 20 g carbohydrate; 6 g protein; 3 g fiber; 39 mg sodium; 329 mg potassium.

Chocolate & Banana

Melt 1 tablespoon semisweet chocolate chips in a small bowl in the microwave. Thinly slice ½ banana and top with the chocolate and 1 tablespoon nonfat vanilla yogurt.

MAKES 1 SERVING.

PER SERVING: 117 calories; 3 g fat (2 g sat, 0 g mono); 0 mg cholesterol; 23 g carbohydrate; 2 g protein; 2 g fiber; 14 mg sodium; 277 mg potassium.

Chocolate-Dipped Strawberries

Melt 2 ounces high-quality dark chocolate over barely simmering water or in the microwave. Dip 12 strawberries in the chocolate.

MAKES 6 SERVINGS.

PER SERVING: 49 calories; 3 g fat (2 g sat, 0 g mono); 0 mg cholesterol; 8 g carbohydrate; 1 g protein; 1 g fiber; 0 mg sodium; 37 mg potassium.

Chocolate Malted Ricotta

Top ¼ cup part-skim ricotta with 1 tablespoon hot cocoa mix and 1 teaspoon malted-milk powder. Stir.

MAKES 1 SERVING.

PER SERVING: 128 calories; 6 g fat (4 g sat, 2 g mono); 21 mg cholesterol; 11 g carbohydrate; 9 g protein; 2 g fiber; 107 mg sodium; 212 mg potassium.

Cinnamon Baked Apples

Preheat oven to 350°F. Create a small well in the center of 4 apples by cutting out the stem and core and leaving the bottom intact. Transfer apples to an 8-by-8-inch glass baking dish. Fill each well with 1 tablespoon brown sugar. Sprinkle ¼ teaspoon cinnamon over apples. Pour 1 cup white wine around the apples, cover with foil and bake until soft, about 1 hour. Let cool before serving.

MAKES 4 SERVINGS.

PER SERVING: 138 calories; 0 g fat (0 g sat, 0 g mono); 0 mg cholesterol; 26 g carbohydrate; 0 g protein; 5 g fiber; 4 mg sodium; 220 mg potassium.

Cinnamon Oranges

With a sharp knife, remove rind and white pith from 4 navel oranges. Cut each into 5 or 6 slices and arrange on 4 plates. Whisk together 2 tablespoons each orange juice and lemon juice, 1 tablespoon sugar and ¼ teaspoon ground cinnamon. Spoon over orange slices.
MAKES 4 SERVINGS.
PER SERVING: 86 calories; 0 g fat (0 g sat, 0 g mono); 0 mg cholesterol; 22 g carbohydrate; 1 g protein; 3 g fiber; 2 mg sodium; 258 mg potassium.

"Cocoa-Nut" Bananas

Place 4 teaspoons unsweetened cocoa powder and 4 teaspoons toasted unsweetened coconut on separate plates. Slice 2 small bananas on the bias, roll each slice in cocoa, shake off the excess, then dip in coconut.
MAKES TK SERVINGS.
PER SERVING: 81 calories; 1 g fat (1 g sat, 0 g mono); 0 mg cholesterol; 19 g carbohydrate; 1 g protein; 2 g fiber; 5 mg sodium; 273 mg potassium.

Farmer's Cheese & Strawberries

Top 1 cup sliced fresh strawberries with ¼ cup farmer's cheese.
MAKES 1 SERVING.
PER SERVING: 153 calories; 6 g fat (3 g sat, 0 g mono); 20 mg cholesterol; 13 g carbohydrate; 11 g protein; 3 g fiber; 242 mg sodium; 254 mg potassium.

Frosted Grapes

Wash and pat dry 2 cups seedless grapes. Freeze 45 minutes. Let stand for 2 minutes at room temperature before serving.
MAKES 4 SERVINGS.
PER SERVING: 55 calories; 0 g fat (0 g sat, 0 g mono); 0 mg cholesterol; 14 g carbohydrate; 1 g protein; 1 g fiber; 2 mg sodium; 153 mg potassium.

Gingered Peach Gratin

Halve and pit 4 peaches. Place the peaches cut-side up in a shallow 1-quart baking dish. Simmer ⅓ cup sugar, ¼ cup lemon juice, 2 tablespoons water and ½ teaspoon ground ginger. Pour over the peaches and sprinkle with 4 crushed gingersnaps. Bake 15 to 20 minutes, or until the peaches are tender and the syrup is thickened.
MAKES 4 SERVINGS.
PER SERVING: 168 calories; 1 g fat (0 g sat, 0 g mono); 0 mg cholesterol; 42 g carbohydrate; 1 g protein; 2 g fiber; 46 mg sodium; 306 mg potassium.

Grilled Peach Sundaes

Preheat grill to high. Cut 2 peaches in half and remove the pits. Brush with canola oil. Grill until tender. Place 2 peach halves in each bowl and top with a scoop of nonfat vanilla frozen yogurt or fruit sorbet and toasted unsweetened coconut.
MAKES 2 SERVINGS.
PER SERVING: 154 calories; 4 g fat (2 g sat, 2 g mono); 0 mg cholesterol; 28 g carbohydrate; 4 g protein; 2 g fiber; 41 mg sodium; 319 mg potassium.

Mini Ice Cream Sandwiches

Top 2 small vanilla-snap cookies with 1 tablespoon each sorbet or frozen yogurt. Top with 2 more cookies. Freeze sandwiches for at least 30 minutes to firm up. Can be wrapped and stored for 1 week.
MAKES 1 SERVING.
PER SERVING: 127 calories; 3 g fat (0 g sat, 0 g mono); 0 mg cholesterol; 24 g carbohydrate; 2 g protein; 2 g fiber; 94 mg sodium; 25 mg potassium.

Pina Colada Yogurt Parfait

Top ⅓ cup reduced-fat vanilla yogurt with ½ cup crushed canned pineapple or ½ cup canned mandarin oranges and 1 tablespoon toasted coconut.
MAKES 1 SERVING.
PER SERVING (with pineapple): 155 calories; 3 g fat (3 g sat, 0 g mono); 4 mg cholesterol; 28 g carbohydrate; 5 g protein; 2 g fiber; 57 mg sodium; 325 mg potassium.

PER SERVING (with oranges): 133 calories; 3 g fat (3 g sat, 0 g mono); 4 mg cholesterol; 22 g carbohydrate; 5 g protein; 1 g fiber; 60 mg sodium; 333 mg potassium.

Pineapple-Coconut Frappe

Blend 1½ cups chopped pineapple, 1 cup low-fat milk, ⅓ cup "lite" coconut milk and 10 ice cubes in a blender until frothy.
MAKES **2** SERVINGS.
PER SERVING: **143** calories; 4 g fat (3 g sat, 1 g mono); 8 mg cholesterol; 23 g carbohydrate; 6 g protein; 2 g fiber; 78 mg sodium; 134 mg potassium.

Pistachio Chocolate Pudding

Top a prepared low-fat chocolate pudding snack cup with 1 tablespoon chopped pistachios.
MAKES **1** SERVING.
PER SERVING: **147** calories; 4 g fat (1 g sat, 2 g mono); 2 mg cholesterol; 25 g carbohydrate; 5 g protein; 2 g fiber; 193 mg sodium; 318 mg potassium.

Quick "Cheesecake"

Spread 4 whole-wheat graham crackers with 1 tablespoon part-skim ricotta cheese and 2 teaspoons jam.
MAKES **1** SERVING.
PER SERVING: **239** calories; 6 g fat (2 g sat, 1 g mono); 10 mg cholesterol; 42 g carbohydrate; 7 g protein; 2 g fiber; 259 mg sodium; 39 mg potassium.

Raspberry-Mango Sundae

Puree ½ cup thawed frozen raspberries, 1 tablespoon sugar and ¼ teaspoon lemon juice in a blender. Serve over scoops of nonfat vanilla frozen yogurt with diced mango and chopped toasted nuts.
MAKES **2** SERVINGS.
PER SERVING: **167** calories; 2 g fat (0 g sat, 2 g mono); 0 mg cholesterol; 35 g carbohydrate; 4 g protein; 2 g fiber; 41 mg sodium; 210 mg potassium.

Roasted Plums

Halve and pit 1½ pounds plums. Place skin-side down in a 9-by-13-inch baking dish. Sprinkle with ⅓ cup sugar and 2 tablespoons lemon juice; bake for 30 to 40 minutes, or until juices are thickened and plums are tender, shaking pan occasionally to distribute juices. Stir in 1 tablespoon brandy and 1 teaspoon grated lemon zest.

MAKES **4** SERVINGS.
PER SERVING: **164** calories; 0 g fat (0 g sat, 0 g mono); 0 mg cholesterol; 41 g carbohydrate; 1 g protein; 2 g fiber; 0 mg sodium; 292 mg potassium.

Spiced Hot Chocolate

Prepare 4 cups hot cocoa with 1% milk. Stir in ½ teaspoon freshly grated nutmeg and ½ teaspoon chili powder. Pour into 4 mugs and garnish each with a cinnamon stick.
MAKES **4** SERVINGS.
PER SERVING: **175** calories; 4 g fat (2 g sat, 1 g mono); 12 mg cholesterol; 30 g carbohydrate; 8 g protein; 1 g fiber; 161 mg sodium; 487 mg potassium.

Tea-Scented Mandarins

Pour ½ cup hot black tea over 2 cups mandarin oranges *or* clementines; drizzle with 2 tablespoons honey and sprinkle with ground cardamom.
MAKES **4** SERVINGS.
PER SERVING: **63** calories; 0 g fat (0 g sat, 0 g mono); 0 mg cholesterol; 16 g carbohydrate; 1 g protein; 2 g fiber; 2 mg sodium; 179 mg potassium.

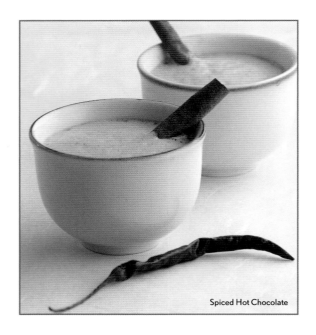

Spiced Hot Chocolate

OTHER RESOURCES

Check out *www.eatingwell.com/diet* to link to all EATINGWELL Diet program resources.

FOR MORE INFORMATION ABOUT WEIGHT MANAGEMENT AND HEALTH:

The Weight-Control Information Network: A national clearinghouse for science-based information on weight control, obesity, physical activity, and related nutritional issues. *http://win.niddk.nih.gov/resources/index.htm*

US Department of Agriculture (USDA) "MyPyramid" Program: Provides general guidelines for a healthy diet and allows you to create a food diary and activity record—with links to nutrition databases for nutrition and calorie information. You can also use an online "MyPyramid Tracker" to record and track your weight for up to a year. *www.mypyramid.gov*

America on the Move Foundation: A national initiative for supporting healthy eating and active living habits, through grass-roots and private partnerships. Best known for encouraging all Americans to strap on pedometers and aim for "10,000 steps per day." *www.americaonthemove.org*; (800) 807-0077

Medline Plus Health Information Database: A service of the National Library of Medicine and the National Institutes of Health, this database supplies links to information on hundreds of health topics, including physical fitness and exercise, and food and nutrition. *http://medlineplus.gov*

National Weight Control Registry: This ongoing survey keeps track of over 5,000 successful "losers" who have maintained a loss of 30 pounds or more for at least one year. Log on for news, research findings, success stories—or to join if you qualify. *http://www.nwcr.ws/*

TO ACCESS ONLINE TOOLS FOR CALCULATING PERSONALIZED WEIGHT AND PHYSICAL ACTIVITY GUIDELINES (USING YOUR PRECISE WEIGHT AND HEIGHT):

Body Mass Index Calculator
National Heart, Lung, and Blood Institute: *http://nhlbisupport.com/bmi/bminojs.htm*

Calories Burned in Physical Activities
Get Moving Calculator, Calorie Control Council: *http://www.caloriecontrol.org/exercalc.html*

FOR NUTRITIONAL COMPOSITION OF VARIOUS FOODS:

Nutritiondata.com lists food label information from packaged foods and includes up-to-date information from fast-food restaurants. *www.nutritiondata.com*

USDA Nutrient Database provides the nutritional composition of thousands of foods from the government's main Nutrient Data Laboratory. *www.nal.usda.gov/fnic/foodcomp/search/*

TO FIND A REGISTERED DIETITIAN:

The American Dietetic Association *www.eatright.org*; (800) 877-1600

BMI CHART

Here is a chart for men and women that gives the BMI for various heights and weights.*
Weight is measured with underwear but no shoes.

BODY MASS INDEX

	21	22	23	24	25	26	27	28	29	30	31
	WEIGHT (in pounds)										
4'10"	100	105	110	115	119	124	129	134	138	143	148
5'0"	107	112	118	123	128	133	138	143	148	153	158
5'1"	111	116	122	127	132	137	143	148	153	158	164
5'3"	118	124	130	135	141	146	152	158	163	169	175
5'5"	126	132	138	144	150	156	162	168	174	180	186
5'7"	134	140	146	153	159	166	172	178	185	191	198
5'9"	142	149	155	162	169	176	182	189	196	203	209
6'0"	150	157	165	172	179	186	193	200	208	215	222
6'1"	159	166	174	182	189	197	204	212	219	227	235
6'3"	168	176	184	192	200	208	216	224	232	240	248

HEIGHT

WHAT DOES YOUR BMI MEAN?

Categories:

Normal weight: BMI = 18.5—24.9. Good for you! Try not to gain weight.

Overweight: BMI = 25—29.9. Do not gain any weight, especially if your waist measurement is high. You need to lose weight if you have two or more risk factors for heart disease and are overweight, or have a high waist measurement.

Obese: BMI = 30 or greater. You need to lose weight. Lose weight slowly—about ½ to 2 pounds a week. See your doctor or a nutritionist if you need help.

Source: Clinical Guidelines on the Identification, Evaluation, and Treatment of Overweight and Obesity in Adults, The Evidence Report, National Heart, Lung, and Blood Institute, in cooperation with the National Institute of Diabetes and Digestive and Kidney Diseases, National Institutes of Health, NIH Publication 98-4083, June 1998.

FOOD DIARY

TODAY'S DATE _____

CALORIE GOAL: _____

Time	Portion	Food or Beverage Description	Calories	Notes

TOTAL CALORIES: _____

Key Foods Checklist (optional)

Nonstarchy Vegetables: ❑ ❑ ❑ ❑ ❑ (❑ ❑ ❑ ❑ ❑)

Fruits: ❑ ❑

Whole Grains: ❑ ❑ ❑

Protein Group: ❑ ❑ ❑ ❑ ❑ (❑)

Calcium-Rich Foods: ❑ ❑

ACTIVITY LOG

TODAY'S DATE _____

CALORIE GOAL: _____

Time	Activity	Duration/ Length	Notes	Calories Burned

TOTAL EXERCISE MINUTES:_____   TOTAL CALORIES BURNED: _____

WEIGHT TRACKER CHART

Use this chart to keep track of your weight changes over time and keep your progress in perspective. Make several copies and keep it handy near your scale. Here's how to customize your chart:

1. Starting with today's date, enter dates along the horizontal bar at the top of the page—using daily or weekly dates, depending on how often you weigh yourself.

2. Write in your current weight at the "starting weight" space along the horizontal axis. (You can leave this blank if you'd rather keep it private!)

3. Plot your daily or weekly weight as points on the chart, connecting the dots with a line.

You'll see firsthand that weight loss never follows a straight line.

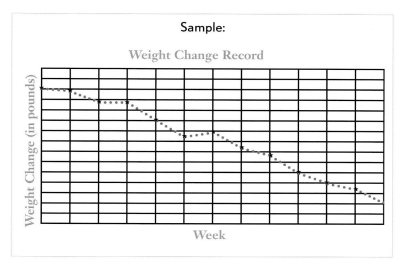

Sample:

Weight Change Record

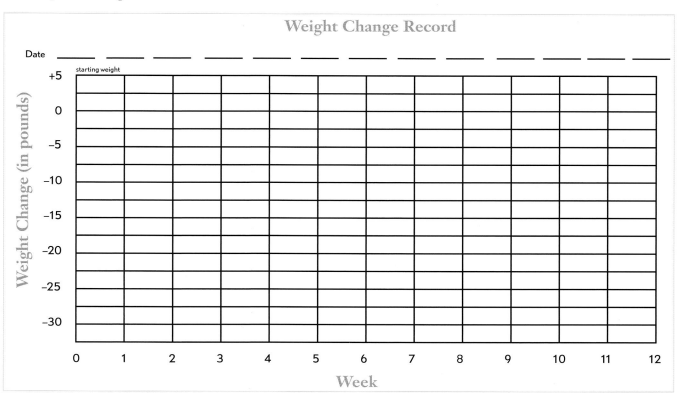

Weight Change Record

CALORIE COUNTERS

	QUANTITY	CALORIES	TOTAL FAT
Cereal and Grain-Based Foods			
Bagel, plain, 3"	0.5 each	73	0
Barley, cooked	0.5 cup	86	1
Biscuit, buttermilk, 2½"	1 each	212	10
Bread, French, slice	1 oz.	78	1
Bread, multigrain,			
low-cal, high-fiber	1 piece	46	1
Bread, oatmeal, slice	1 piece	73	1
Bread, pita, wheat, 6½"	0.5 each	85	1
Bread, rye	1 piece	80	1
Bread, whole-wheat, slice	1 piece	69	1
Breadsticks, sesame, toasted	1 oz.	120	4
Bulgur, whole-wheat	0.5 cup	96	0
Buns, hamburger,			
whole-wheat	1 each	114	2
Couscous, whole-wheat	0.5 cup	140	1
Crackers, graham,			
Honey Maid	1 rectangle	122	3
Crackers, matzo, plain	1 each	112	0
Crackers, Saltine	6 each	77	2
Croutons, seasoned, cubes	0.5 cup	93	4
English muffin, plain	0.5 each	70	1
English muffin, whole-wheat	0.5 each	67	1
Grits, corn, cooked in water	0.5 cup	71	0
Kasha, cooked	0.5 cup	77	1
Oatmeal, instant,			
flavored	0.5 cup	149	1
Oatmeal, cooked in water,			
plain	0.5 cup	74	1
Pasta, macaroni, cooked	0.5 cup	111	1
Pasta, spaghetti, whole-wheat,			
cooked	0.5 cup	87	0
Popcorn, air-popped	2 cup	62	1
Popcorn, popped in oil, salted	2 cup	110	6
Polenta, prepared tube	4 oz.	80	0
Pretzels, tiny twists, fat-free	1 oz.	100	0
Rice, brown, cooked	0.5 cup	109	1
Rice, white, cooked	0.5 cup	103	0
Taco shells, corn	1 each	64	3
Tortilla, corn, 6"	1 each	57	1
Tortilla, whole-wheat	1 each	73	0

	QUANTITY	CALORIES	TOTAL FAT
Condiments, Flavorings & Broths			
Anchovy paste	1 tsp.	40	3
Broth, chicken, canned	1 cup	39	1
Broth, vegetable	1 cup	30	0
Capers	1 Tbsp.	1	0
Dip, sour cream	1 oz.	63	6
Honey	1 tsp.	21	0
Ketchup	1 Tbsp.	15	0
Mayonnaise, reduced-fat	1 Tbsp.	49	5
Mayonnaise, regular	1 Tbsp.	99	11
Mustard, any kind	1 tsp.	3	0
Oil, any kind	1 tsp.	40	5
Olives, black, large, without			
pits, canned	3 each	15	1
Olives, green, stuffed	3 each	12	1
Peanut butter, chunky			
or creamy	1 Tbsp.	94	8
Pickles, kosher dill, spears	1 each	5	0
Relish, pickle, sweet	1 tsp.	7	0
Relish, vegetable	1 tsp.	1	0
Salad dressing, Caesar	2 Tbsp.	155	17
Salad dressing, Caesar,			
low-calorie	2 Tbsp.	33	1
Salad dressing, French	2 Tbsp.	143	14
Salad dressing, honey-			
mustard	2 Tbsp.	102	6
Salad dressing, Italian	2 Tbsp.	86	8
Salad dressing, Italian,			
low-calorie	2 Tbsp.	23	2
Salad dressing,			
mayonnaise type	1 Tbsp.	57	5
Salad dressing, Ranch,			
fat-free	2 Tbsp.	34	1
Salad dressing, Ranch,			
reduced-fat	2 Tbsp.	62	5
Sauce, pesto	1 Tbsp.	78	7
Sauce, soy, low-sodium	1 tsp.	3	0
Sugar	1 tsp.	10	0
Splenda, granular	1 tsp.	2	0
Tomatoes, sun-dried	1 Tbsp.	12	0
Vinegar, distilled	1 tsp.	1	0

Dairy & Eggs	QUANTITY	CALORIES	TOTAL FAT
Butter, unsalted	1 tsp.	33	4
Butter, salted, whipped	1 tsp.	23	3
Buttermilk, low-fat, cultured	1 cup	98	2
Cheese, blue, crumbled	1 oz.	101	8
Cheese, Brie	1 oz.	95	8
Cheese, Cheddar, low-fat, shredded	1 oz.	49	2
Cheese, Cheddar	1 oz.	114	9
Cheese, feta	1 oz.	60	5
Cheese, feta, 50% less fat, 1 1/4" cube	1 oz.	50	3
Cheese, fontina	1 oz.	110	9
Cheese, goat, semisoft	1 oz.	103	8
Cheese, Monterey Jack	1 oz.	106	9
Cheese, mozzarella, part-skim	1 oz.	72	5
Cheese, Parmesan, grated	1 oz.	122	8
Cheese, ricotta, part-skim	0.5 cup	171	10
Cheese, Swiss	1 oz.	108	8
Coffee creamer	1 Tbsp.	20	1
Cottage cheese, 2% fat	0.5 cup	102	2
Cottage cheese, low-fat, low-sodium	0.5 cup	81	1
Cream cheese, soft	1 Tbsp.	50	5
Cream cheese, low-fat	1 Tbsp.	35	3
Egg, large	1 each	78	5
Egg, substitute, liquid	1/4 cup	30	0
Frozen yogurt, vanilla or strawberry, nonfat	0.5 cup	95	0
Milk, whole	1 cup	146	8
Milk, 2%	1 cup	122	5
Milk, 1%	1 cup	110	3
Milk, nonfat/skim	1 cup	83	0
Sour cream	1 Tbsp.	30	3
Sour cream, nonfat	1 Tbsp.	10	0
Soymilk, low-fat	8 oz.	90	2
Soymilk, nonfat	8 oz.	70	0
Yogurt, vanilla, low-fat	6 oz.	145	2
Yogurt, plain, nonfat	6 oz.	95	0

Fish & Seafood	QUANTITY	CALORIES	TOTAL FAT
Catfish, baked or broiled	3 oz.	129	7
Cod, baked or broiled	3 oz.	89	1
Flounder, baked or broiled	3 oz.	100	1
Salmon, baked or broiled	3 oz.	155	7
Salmon, smoked (lox)	1 oz.	43	2
Sardines, no skin or bone, water-canned	1 oz.	62	4
Scallops, baked or broiled	3 oz.	114	3
Shrimp, cooked	3 oz.	84	1
Tilapia, baked or broiled	3 oz.	109	2
Trout, baked or broiled	3 oz.	162	7
Tuna, baked or broiled	3 oz.	156	5
Tuna, light, canned with water, drained	3 oz.	99	1

Fruit	QUANTITY	CALORIES	TOTAL FAT
Apples, small, fresh	1 each	62	0
Applesauce, unsweetened	0.5 cup	52	0
Apricots, fresh or dried	1 each	17	0
Banana, 6"-6 7/8" long	1 each	90	0
Blackberries, fresh	1 cup	62	1
Blueberries, fresh	1 cup	83	0
Cherries, dried	1 oz.	62	0
Cherries, fresh	1 cup	91	0
Coconut, dried, unsweetened	1 Tbsp.	31	3
Coconut milk, "lite"	0.5 cup	96	8
Cranberries, Craisins	1 oz.	92	0
Dates, dried	1 oz.	79	0
Fruit cocktail	0.5 cup	80	0
Grapefruit, 3 1/2"	0.5 each	32	0
Grapes, fresh	1 cup	110	0
Juice, apple	0.5 cup	58	0
Juice, cranberry	0.5 cup	68	0
Juice, lemon, fresh	1 Tbsp.	4	0
Juice, orange	0.5 cup	56	0
Juice, tomato	0.5 cup	20	0
Juice, vegetable	0.5 cup	23	0
Kiwi, fresh, medium	1 oz.	17	0
Mango, fresh, whole	0.5 each	67	0
Melon, cantaloupe, cubes	1 cup	54	0
Melon, honeydew, cubes	1 cup	61	0
Nectarines, fresh, medium	1 each	60	0
Oranges, fresh, medium	1 each	62	0
Papaya, fresh, cubes	1 cup	55	0
Peaches, fresh, medium	1 each	38	0
Pears, fresh, Bartlett, medium	1 each	96	0
Pineapple, fresh, diced	1 cup	70	0
Plums, fresh	1 each	30	0
Prunes, dried	1 oz.	77	0
Raisins, seedless	0.5 cup	108	0
Raspberries, fresh	1 cup	64	1

	QUANTITY	CALORIES	TOTAL FAT
Rhubarb, fresh, diced	1 cup	13	0
Strawberries, fresh	1 cup	49	0
Tangerines, fresh, medium	1 each	45	0
Watermelon, fresh, diced	1 cup	46	0

Meats and Poultry

	QUANTITY	CALORIES	TOTAL FAT
Bacon, cooked	1 piece	29	2
Beef, London broil, broiled	3 oz.	165	7
Beef, ground or patty, broiled, 10% fat	3 oz.	185	10
Beef, ground or patty, broiled, 15% fat	3 oz.	213	13
Beef, filet mignon, lean, broiled	3 oz.	164	7
Beef, strip steak, lean, broiled	3 oz.	174	8
Beef, top sirloin or round steak, broiled	3 oz.	150	4
Canadian bacon, serving	1 oz.	35	1
Chicken, rotisserie-cooked	3 oz.	157	7
Chicken, breast, oven-roasted, fat-free, sliced	1 oz.	22	0
Chicken, breast, no skin, roasted	3 oz.	140	3
Chicken, thigh, no skin, roasted	3 oz.	178	9
Chicken, tenders, cooked	3 oz.	105	0
Crab, canned	3 oz.	84	1
Crab, king, leg, baked or broiled	3 oz.	117	5
Ham, deli, extra-lean, sliced	1 oz.	31	1
Pork, prosciutto, sliced	1 oz.	61	3
Pork, tenderloin chop, broiled	3 oz.	171	7
Pork, tenderloin, lean, roasted	3 oz.	139	4
Salami, sliced	1 oz.	73	6
Sausage, turkey, cooked	3 oz.	167	9
Turkey, light meat, no skin, roasted	3 oz.	134	3
Turkey, breast cutlets, cooked	3 oz.	120	1
Turkey, breast, deli, sliced	1 oz.	27	0
Turkey, ground, 99% fat-free, cooked	3 oz.	120	2

Nuts, Seeds and Beans

	QUANTITY	CALORIES	TOTAL FAT
Nuts, almonds, dry-roasted	1 oz.	169	15
Nuts, cashews, dry-roasted	1 oz.	163	13
Nuts, peanuts, dry-roasted	1 oz.	166	14
Nuts, pecans, dry-roasted	1 oz.	201	21
Nuts, pine (pignoli), dried	0.25 cup	229	23
Nuts, pistachio, shelled	1 oz.	158	13
Nuts, walnuts, dried, halves	1 oz.	185	18
Seeds, pumpkin/squash, kernels	1 oz.	153	13
Seeds, sesame	1 Tbsp.	59	6
Seeds, sunflower, kernels, toasted	1 oz.	175	16
Beans, baked	0.5 cup	118	1
Beans, black, cooked	0.5 cup	331	1
Beans, butter, cooked	0.5 cup	70	0
Beans, chickpea, cooked	0.5 cup	143	1
Beans, kidney, cooked	0.5 cup	105	1
Beans, lentils, cooked	0.5 cup	115	0
Beans, navy, cooked	0.5 cup	148	1
Beans, pinto, cooked	0.5 cup	103	1
Beans, white, cooked	0.5 cup	153	0
Soybeans, green (edamame), cooked	0.5 cup	127	6
Tofu	0.5 cup	94	6

Vegetables

	QUANTITY	CALORIES	TOTAL FAT
Artichoke hearts, canned with water	0.5 cup	61	0
Arugula, leaves, fresh	1 cup	7	0
Asparagus spears, fresh, 5¼"-7" long	0.5 cup	23	0
Avocado, fresh	0.25 each	80	7
Beans, green, fresh or cooked	0.5 cup	17	0
Bean sprouts, mung, cooked	0.5 cup	13	0
Beets, slices, cooked	0.5 cup	26	0
Belgian endive, fresh	1 cup	15	0
Broccoli, florets, fresh	0.5 cup	10	0
Brussels sprouts, fresh	0.5 cup	19	0
Cabbage, bok choy, cooked	0.5 cup	10	0
Cabbage, cooked, red or green	0.5 cup	17	0

	QUANTITY	CALORIES	TOTAL FAT		QUANTITY	CALORIES	TOTAL FAT
Carrots, fresh, chopped	0.5 cup	26	0	Peppers, fresh bell,			
Cauliflower, florets, fresh	0.5 cup	28	0	red or green	0.5 cup	25	0
Celery, fresh, diced	0.5 cup	8	0	Potatoes, boiled	0.5 cup	98	0
Corn, kernels, fresh				Radishes, fresh, sliced	0.5 cup	18	0
or cooked	0.5 cup	66	1	Salad, mixed greens, fresh	1 cup	9	0
Cucumber slices, fresh	0.5 cup	8	0	Spinach, baby, fresh	1 cup	6	0
Eggplant, cooked	0.5 cup	17	0	Spinach, steamed	0.5 cup	21	0
Fennel, bulb, fresh	0.5 cup	35	0	Squash, butternut,			
Kale, cooked	0.5 cup	18	0	fresh, cubes	0.5 cup	54	0
Leeks, cooked	0.5 cup	16	0	Squash, summer,			
Lettuce, fresh, any type	1 cup	7	0	all types, fresh	0.5 cup	18	0
Mushrooms, fresh	0.5 cup	11	0	Sweet potatoes, cooked	0.5 cup	122	0
Okra, cooked	0.5 cup	26	0	Swiss chard, cooked	0.5 cup	18	0
Onion, fresh	0.5 cup	46	0	Tomatoes, fresh	0.5 cup	20	0
Peas, green, cooked	0.5 cup	55	0	Tomatoes, stewed	0.5 cup	30	0
Peas, snow or sugar snap,				Turnips, cooked	0.5 cup	18	0
cooked	0.5 cup	35	0	Watercress, fresh, chopped	1 cup	4	0

" Finish each day and be done with it. You have done what you could; some blunders and absurdities have crept in; forget them as soon as you can. Tomorrow is a new day; you shall begin it serenely and with too high a spirit to be encumbered with your old nonsense. "

RALPH WALDO EMERSON

THE EATINGWELL PANTRY

OILS, VINEGARS & CONDIMENTS
- Extra-virgin olive oil for cooking and salad dressings
- Canola oil for cooking and baking
- Flavorful nut and seed oils for salad dressings and stir-fry seasonings: toasted sesame oil, walnut oil
- Butter, preferably unsalted. Store in the freezer if you use infrequently.
- Reduced-fat mayonnaise
- Vinegars: balsamic, red-wine, white-wine, rice, cider
- Asian condiments and flavorings: reduced-sodium soy sauce, fish sauce, hoisin sauce, mirin, oyster sauce, chile-garlic sauce, curry paste
- Kalamata olives, green olives
- Dijon mustard
- Capers
- Ketchup
- Barbecue sauce
- Worcestershire sauce

FLAVORINGS
- Kosher salt, coarse sea salt, fine salt
- Black peppercorns
- Onions
- Fresh garlic
- Fresh ginger
- Anchovies or anchovy paste for flavoring pasta sauces and salad dressings
- Dried herbs: bay leaves, dill, crumbled dried sage, thyme, oregano, tarragon, Italian seasoning blend
- Spices: allspice (whole berries or ground), caraway seeds, chili powder, cinnamon sticks, ground cinnamon, coriander seeds, ground coriander, cumin seeds, ground cumin, curry powder, ground ginger, dry mustard, nutmeg, paprika, cayenne pepper, crushed red pepper, turmeric

- Lemons, limes, oranges. The zest is as valuable as the juice. Organic fruit is recommended when you use a lot of zest.
- Granulated sugar
- Brown sugar
- Honey
- Pure maple syrup
- Unsweetened cocoa powder, natural and/or Dutch-processed
- Bittersweet chocolate, semisweet chocolate chips

CANNED GOODS &
BOTTLED ITEMS
- Canned tomatoes, tomato paste
- Reduced-sodium chicken broth, beef broth and/or vegetable broth
- Clam juice
- "Lite" coconut milk for Asian curries and soups
- Canned beans: cannellini beans, great northern beans, chickpeas, black beans, red kidney beans, pinto beans
- Canned lentils
- Chunk light tuna, salmon and sardines

GRAINS & LEGUMES
- Whole-wheat flour and whole-wheat pastry flour (Store opened packages in the refrigerator or freezer.)
- All-purpose flour
- Assorted whole-wheat pastas
- Brown rice and instant brown rice
- Pearl barley, quick-cooking barley
- Rolled oats
- Whole-wheat couscous
- Bulgur
- Dried lentils
- Yellow cornmeal
- Plain dry breadcrumbs
- Wild rice

NUTS, SEEDS & FRUITS
- Walnuts
- Pecans
- Almonds
- Hazelnuts
- Dry-roasted unsalted peanuts
- Pine nuts
- Sesame seeds
    (Store opened packages of nuts and seeds in the refrigerator or freezer.)
- Natural peanut butter
- Tahini
- Assorted dried fruits, such as apricots, prunes, cherries, cranberries, dates, figs, raisins

REFRIGERATOR BASICS
- Low-fat milk or soymilk
- Low-fat or nonfat plain yogurt and/or vanilla yogurt
- Reduced-fat sour cream
- Good-quality Parmesan cheese and/or Romano cheese
- Sharp Cheddar cheese
- Eggs (large). Keep them on hand for fast omelets and frittatas.
- Orange juice
- Dry white wine. If you wish, substitute nonalcoholic wine.
- Water-packed tofu

FREEZER BASICS
- Fruit-juice concentrates (orange, apple, pineapple)
- Frozen vegetables: edamame (soybeans), peas, spinach, broccoli, bell pepper and onion mix, corn, chopped onions, small whole onions, uncooked hash browns
- Frozen berries
- Italian turkey sausage and sliced prosciutto to flavor fast pasta sauces
- Low-fat vanilla ice cream or frozen yogurt for impromptu desserts

COOKING TIPS

To **clean leeks:** Trim off fuzzy root and dark green stems. With a sharp knife, cut several incisions in the leek's stem end to open it up like a fan. Soak in water for several minutes, then swish to dislodge dirt. Repeat until no grit remains.

To **hard-boil eggs:** Place eggs in a single layer in a saucepan; cover with water. Bring to a simmer over medium-high heat. Reduce heat to low and cook at the barest simmer for 10 minutes. Remove from heat, pour out hot water and run a constant stream of cold water over the eggs until completely cooled.

To **oil a grill rack**, oil a folded paper towel, hold it with tongs and rub it over the rack. (Do not use cooking spray on a hot grill.)

To **poach chicken breasts:** Place boneless, skinless chicken breasts in a medium skillet or saucepan and add enough water to cover; bring to a boil. Cover, reduce heat to low and simmer gently until the chicken is cooked through and no longer pink in the middle, 10 to 12 minutes.

To **skin a salmon fillet:** Place salmon fillet on a clean cutting board, skin-side down. Starting at the tail end, slip the blade of a long knife between the fish flesh and the skin, holding down firmly with your other hand. Gently push the blade along at a 30° angle, separating the fillet from the skin without cutting through either.

To **toast chopped nuts & seeds:** Cook in a small dry skillet over medium-low heat, stirring constantly, until fragrant and lightly browned, 2 to 4 minutes.

INGREDIENT NOTES

Buttermilk substitution: In place of fresh buttermilk you can use buttermilk powder, such as Saco Buttermilk Blend; look for it in the baking section or with the powdered milk in most supermarkets. Or make "sour milk": mix 1 tablespoon lemon juice (or vinegar) to 1 cup milk.

Lavash is a soft, thin flatbread commonly used in Armenian or Iranian cuisine. Find it in well-stocked supermarkets or Middle Eastern specialty markets.

Potatoes, precooked and diced, can be found in the refrigerated section of the produce and/or dairy department of the supermarket. (*Alternatively, boil potatoes until they can just be pierced with a fork but are not completely tender. Let cool slightly, then dice.*)

Rice vinegar (or rice-wine vinegar) is mild, slightly sweet vinegar made from fermented rice. Find it in the Asian section of supermarkets and specialty stores.

Shao Hsing (or Shaoxing) is a seasoned rice wine. It is available in most Asian specialty markets and some larger supermarkets in the Asian section. Dry sherry is an acceptable substitute.

Sherry: The "cooking sherry" sold in many supermarkets can be surprisingly high in sodium. We prefer dry to medium sherry, sold with other fortified wines in your wine or liquor store.

Whole-wheat pastry flour is milled from soft wheat. It contains less gluten than regular whole-wheat flour and helps ensure a tender result in delicate baked goods while providing the nutritional benefits of whole grains. Look for it in the natural-foods section of large supermarkets and natural-foods stores. Sources include King Arthur Flour, (800) 827-6836, www.bakerscatalogue.com, and Bob's Red Mill, (800) 349-2173, www.bobsredmill.com.

SUBJECT INDEX

RECIPE INDEX

Our thanks to the fine cooks whose work has appeared in EATINGWELL Magazine. (*Page numbers in italics indicate photographs.*)

CONGRATULATIONS! You've made that first step toward healthy, sustainable weight loss. Now, visit us at *www.eatingwell.com/diet* to:

- Order your personal EatingWell Diet Food Diary
- Review the 7 Steps to Healthy & Permanent Weight Loss
- Download our popular EatingWell Diet worksheets
- Learn practical, self-support techniques to achieve lifelong weight loss
- Search more than 1,000 recipes in the EatingWell.com Recipe Library
- Stay up-to-date on the latest food and nutrition news
- Get support from experts and fellow EatingWell enthusiasts
- Subscribe to EatingWell Magazine

EatingWell.com, our free website, and EATINGWELL Magazine will help you stay motivated and make it easy for you and your family to enjoy simple, delicious meals every day.

Take the next steps at: **WWW.EATINGWELL.COM/DIET**

OTHER EATINGWELL BOOKS
(available at *www.eatingwell.com/shop*):

The Essential EatingWell Cookbook
(The Countryman Press, 2004)
ISBN-13: 978-0-88150-701-0 (softcover)

The EatingWell Diabetes Cookbook
(The Countryman Press, 2005)
ISBN-13: 978-0-88150-633-4 (hardcover)

The EatingWell Healthy in a Hurry Cookbook
(The Countryman Press, 2006)
ISBN-13: 978-0-88150-687-7 (hardcover)

EatingWell Serves 2
(The Countryman Press, 2006)
ISBN-13: 978-0-88150-723-2 (hardcover)